Fast Facts for the WOUND CARE NURSE: Practical Wound Management in a Nutshell (*Kifer*)

Fast Facts About EKGs FOR NURSES: The Rules of Identifying EKGs in a Nutshell (*Landrum*)

Fast Facts for the CRITICAL CARE NURSE: Critical Care Nursing in a Nutshell (*Landrum*)

Fast Facts for the TRAVEL NURSE: Travel Nursing in a Nutshell (*Landrum*)

Fast Facts for the SCHOOL NURSE: School Nursing in a Nutshell, 2e (*Loschiavo*)

Fast Facts About CURRICULUM DEVELOPMENT IN NURSING: How to Develop & Evaluate Educational Programs in a Nutshell (*McCoy, Anema*)

Fast Facts for DEMENTIA CARE: What Nurses Need to Know in a Nutshell (*Miller*)

Fast Facts for HEALTH PROMOTION IN NURSING: Promoting Wellness in a Nutshell (*Miller*)

Fast Facts for STROKE CARE NURSING: An Expert Guide in a Nutshell (*Morrison*)

Fast Facts for the MEDICAL OFFICE NURSE: What You Really Need to Know in a Nutshell (*Richmeier*)

Fast Facts for the PEDIATRIC NURSE: An Orientation Guide in a Nutshell (*Rupert, Young*)

Fast Facts About the GYNECOLOGICAL EXAM FOR NURSE PRACTITIONERS: Conducting the GYN Exam in a Nutshell (*Secor, Fantasia*)

Fast Facts for the STUDENT NURSE: Nursing Student Success in a Nutshell (*Stabler-Haas*)

Fast Facts for CAREER SUCCESS IN NURSING: Making the Most of Mentoring in a Nutshell (*Vance*)

Fast Facts for the TRIAGE NURSE: An Orientation and Care Guide in a Nutshell (*Visser, Montejano, Grossman*)

Fast Facts for DEVELOPING A NURSING ACADEMIC PORTFOLIO: What You Really Need to Know in a Nutshell (*Wittmann-Price*)

Fast Facts for the HOSPICE NURSE: A Concise Guide to End-of-Life Care (*Wright*)

Fast Facts for the CLASSROOM NURSING INSTRUCTOR: Classroom Teaching in a Nutshell (*Yoder-Wise, Kowalski*)

Forthcoming FAST FACTS Books

Fast Facts About PTSD: A Clinician's Guide to Post-Traumatic Stress Disorder in a Nutshell (*Adams*)

Fast Facts on COMBATING NURSE BULLYING, INCIVILITY, AND WORKPLACE VIOLENCE: What Nurses Need to Know in a Nutshell (*Ciocco*)

Fast Facts for TESTING AND EVALUATION IN NURSING: Teaching Skills in a Nutshell (*Dusaj*)

Fast Facts About the NURSING PROFESSION: Historical Perspectives in a Nutshell (*Hunt*)

Fast Facts for the CLINICAL NURSING INSTRUCTOR: Nursing Student Success in a Nutshell, 3e (*Kan, Stabler-Haas*)

Fast Facts for the CRITICAL CARE NURSE: Critical Care Nursing in Nutshell, 2e (*Landrum*)

Fast Facts About NURSING PATIENTS WITH MENTAL ILLNESS (MI): What RNs, NPs, and New Psych Nurses Need to Know (*Marshall*)

Fast Facts About the GYNECOLOGIC EXAM: A Professional Guide for NPs, PAs, and Midwives, 2e (*Secor, Fantasia*)

FAST FACTS for
the **ER NURSE**

Jennifer R. Buettner, RN, CEN, currently serves as the nurse educator for the emergency department (ED) at DeKalb Medical Center at Hillandale, Lithonia, Georgia. In this role, Mrs. Buettner works to advance the careers of emergency nurses through education and evidence-based practice. She finds great joy in helping others grow professionally and cultivate their inner gifts and talents. She has developed ED orientation processes and education courses for several local hospitals in the Atlanta, Georgia, area. In her 17 years of ED nursing experience, she has spent several years precepting new emergency nurses and has served as a legal nurse consultant. Mrs. Buettner holds certifications in basic disaster life support (BDLS), advanced disaster life support (ADLS), and as a certified emergency nurse (CEN), and serves as an advanced cardiac life support (ACLS), pediatric advanced life support (PALS), and cardiopulmonary resuscitation (CPR) instructor. She is a course coordinator for the trauma nursing core course (TNCC) and emergency nursing pediatric course (ENPC). She is a current member of the Emergency Nurses Association and an advocate for the Board Certified Emergency Nursing exam. She received the Faculty Award from the Virginia Beach School of Practical Nursing, for the graduate who "has achieved excellence in both the academic and clinical settings and who best exemplifies the total integration of program philosophy to professional performance" (March 1999). In 2010, Mrs. Buettner was nominated as nurse of the year by the *Atlanta Journal-Constitution*. She was a finalist for the 2016 Atlanta March of Dime's Nurse of the Year Award. Her passion to teach and mentor new ED nurses led her to create an original ED orientation manual made specifically for new emergency nurses and their preceptors.

FAST FACTS for the **ER NURSE**

Emergency Department Orientation in a Nutshell

Third Edition

Jennifer R. Buettner, RN, CEN

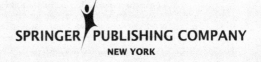

SPRINGER PUBLISHING COMPANY
NEW YORK

Springer Publishing Company, LLC
11 West 42nd Street
New York, NY 10036
www.springerpub.com

Acquisitions Editor: Elizabeth Nieginski
Senior Production Editor: Kris Parrish
Compositor: Westchester Publishing Services

ISBN: 978-0-8261-1859-2
e-book ISBN: 978-0-8261-1864-6

17 18 19 20 / 5 4 3 2 1

Library of Congress Cataloging-in-Publication Data

Names: Buettner, Jennifer R., author.
Title: Fast facts for the ER nurse : emergency department orientation in a nutshell / Jennifer R. Buettner.
Other titles: Fast facts for the emergency room nurse | Fast facts (Springer Publishing Company)
Description: Third edition. | New York, NY : Springer Publishing Company, [2017] | Series: Fast facts | Includes bibliographical references and index.
Identifiers: LCCN 2016059892 | ISBN 9780826118592 (hardcopy: alk. paper) | ISBN 9780826118646 (e-book) | ISBN 9780829119858 (PowerPoints) | ISBN 9780826119797 (audiobook)
Subjects: | MESH: Emergencies—nursing | Emergency Nursing—methods | Critical Illness—nursing
Classification: LCC RT120.E4 | NLM WY 154.2 | DDC 616.02/5—dc23
LC record available at https://lccn.loc.gov/2016059892

Printed in the United States of America by Gasch Printing.

This book is dedicated to ED nurses everywhere. May you always thirst for knowledge, but let your cup be full of strength, grace, compassion, mercy, and love. May God bless your hearts and hands as you touch so many patients in need every day.

Contents

Preface

This is a book designed for *real* emergency department (ED) nurses by a *real* ED nurse. It is a quick reference book intended to aid your day-to-day ED orientation process with your preceptor and to guide you through the most common illnesses seen in the ED. This book does not cover basic anatomy and physiology, advanced cardiovascular life support, pediatric advanced life support, or the trauma nurse core course. The information in this book is compiled from basic ED knowledge and the sources used are considered reliable.

There are several points to take into consideration in referencing this book. First, all listed interventions that go beyond the scope of nursing practice should be followed as ordered by the ED provider. Second, the term "provider" in this book could be a physician (MD or DO), a nurse practitioner (NP), or a physician assistant (PA), who is qualified to provide such ED patient care. In most cases, interventions that go beyond the usual scope of nursing practice have been introduced using "Anticipate an order to" followed by a list of possible provider orders. As always, it is the nurse's responsibility to check any noted medication dosages or treatments to ensure that all are current, recommended, and accepted practices.

After reading this book, you will become the "Jack of all illnesses." So, put on your running shoes, keep a stash of dark chocolates, and when all else fails, practice unreasonable happiness. One thing is for sure: Just when you think you have seen it all, your next patient will come in!

Each chapter includes a brief introduction; an outline of materials, equipment, and drugs with which you should become familiar; a list of diagnoses that includes definitions, causes, signs and symptoms, and interventions; a feature titled "Fast Facts in a Nutshell" that provides quick summaries of important points; and question-and-answer boxes for your review. The appendices at the end of the book include abbreviations, common lab values, EKG rhythms, and frequently used ED medications—information that should become second nature to all ED personnel.

There are two ways to use this book. You can review the book cover to cover, or you can use the skills check-off sheets in Appendix F and review the appropriate chapters.

Jennifer R. Buettner

Acknowledgments

I could not do what I do without the support of my loving husband, Nick, and our friends and family. Nevertheless, the base of my emergency nursing foundation was built by my first preceptor, Linda Whitt, BSN, RN. I thank her for her patience, sharing her wealth of knowledge, and setting a prime example of a truly humble, wise, and compassionate nurse. I cannot forget my second preceptor, Walter McCracken, RN, whose pearls of wisdom can be found in no book. Special thanks go to my editor, Elizabeth Nieginski, and the Springer Publishing team for bringing my thoughts and ideas for this book to life. I am truly honored to be a part of a dedicated, knowledgeable, and compassionate ED leadership team, including; Shunda Harper, MSN, RN, Tamiko Smith, MSN, FNP-C, Sealena White, BSN, RN, and Natasha Allen, RN, CEN—I thank you for mentoring, supporting, and inspiring me even on my weakest days! To all my friends and colleagues who have inspired me and molded me into the ED nurse I am today, I am forever grateful.

Last, but not least, I would like to thank the nurse and good friend who inspired me to write this book and never stopped believing in me, Nichole Lunsford Howell, BSN, RN.

Above all, my faith has sustained me through all my endeavors; I give thanks and glory to God for all of His gifts and blessings.

I would like to acknowledge the work of the following individuals in offering their professional opinions and reviewing the content in this book for accuracy.

Acknowledgments

REVIEWERS OF THIS EDITION

Natasha Allen, RN, CEN
R. Bruce Bessey, MD, FAAP
Nancy Capponi, MSN, RN, CEN, CCRN
Julie Espinosa, MSN, RN, CEN, EMT-P
Paula Funderberke, MS, RN, CEN, CPEN, CNS-BC
Shunda L. Harper, MSN, RN
Nichole Lunsford Howell, BSN, RN
Chanique Kelley, MSN, RN, CEN
Paul Olander, MSW, JD, LCSW, CCM, NBCCH, RRT-P
Laura K. Phillips, MSN, RN
Joshua W. Shoemaker, PharmD, BCPS
Tamiko Smith, MSN, FNP-C
Sealena White, BSN, RN

PREVIOUS EDITION REVIEWERS

Teresa M. Campo, DNP, RN, NP-C
Joanne Davis, DMD
Kurtis Davis, DMD
Cyndi Griffith, BSN, RN
Heather Hall, MD
Shunda L. Harper, MSN, RN
Nichole Lunsford, BSN, RN
Laura K. Phillips, BSN, RN

1

Tips on Surviving ED Nursing

Even if you love working in the emergency department (ED), it can be tough at times. The ED is particularly stressful because you care for a broad spectrum of patients in a fast-paced, critical environment. So, not only do you need to be extremely knowledgeable, you also need to be organized, calm, and fast on your feet. Everyone knows that the nurses are the very heart of the ED. Your patients rely on you. But **to take care of others, you first need to take care of yourself,** physically, mentally, and spiritually. This chapter includes a checklist of stress symptoms and a list of simple methods for coping with those pressures.

During this part of your orientation, you will learn:

- How to recognize the symptoms of stress on the job
- Basic techniques you can use on the job to alleviate that stress

SYMPTOMS OF STRESS

It is true that ED nurses are sometimes referred to as "adrenaline junkies." However, one cannot function on adrenaline alone. Severe stress and anxiety on the job are harmful to you and your patients. So learn to recognize the signs and symptoms: severe muscle tension, fatigue, irritability, flight or fight response, tachycardia, tachypnea, weakness, sweating, feeling helpless, anger, tearfulness, urinary urgency, diarrhea, dry mouth, insomnia, difficulty in problem solving, feeling overwhelmed, and decreased appetite.

Fast Facts in a Nutshell

To take care of others, you first need to take care of yourself.

TECHNIQUES FOR RELIEVING STRESS

- Take a moment, close your eyes, and take some deep cleansing breaths. Breathe in through your nose as you count to five. Then exhale slowly through your mouth as you count to five, and that's it. Breathing exercises increase oxygen to your brain and are a fast, simple way to relieve stress anytime, anywhere.
- Stay hydrated. Keep a water bottle with you at work. Staying hydrated is an easy way to stay healthy.
- Focus on the positives. When you have a complaint, spend your energy finding a solution rather than complaining. You need all the energy you can get, so use it to resolve stressful problems.
- Schedule time in your regular work week for rest and rejuvenation. Consider ways to rest physically, mentally, and spirituality.
- Listen to upbeat energizing music on the way to work so that the melody will repeat itself in your head all day. "Whistle while you work." Singing or humming is a good way to relieve stress.
- Keep a stash of *dark* chocolates: They are actually a source of energy and antioxidants. Dark chocolate not only boosts your immune system, but it also seems to make people happy. It works well on any grumpy coworkers too, so do not forget to share.
- Introduce yourself to patients when you enter a room. Keeping the patients informed of who you are and what you are going to be doing relieves their stress.
- Wear a well-made, comfortable pair of shoes. Eight to 12 hours of painful swollen feet will only add to your stress.
- Recognize that it is perfectly normal to feel anxious during a code (e.g., cardiac/pulmonary arrest). Only time and training will help you cope with the anxiety felt when performing advanced cardiovascular life supportive treatments.

- Do not think or act as if you know it all. Medicine is constantly changing. No matter how much ED experience you have, you can still learn something new every day. Seek frequent feedback from your leaders and learn from other high-performing colleagues.
- Keep the following in your pocket every day: trauma shears, hemostats, tape, pen, calculator (with list of ED intravenous drips and doses taped to back), and this book. Being prepared will reduce stress and anxiety.
- Invest in a good pair of support hose and do leg exercises. Most nurses develop varicose veins. It is hard to take good care of your patients when your legs ache and have poor circulation.
- Ask or look up any medications about which you are unsure. There are numerous medication routes and doses to memorize. Looking them up or asking will help you learn them and keep your patients safe and free of medication errors.
- Keep your uniforms clean, to save yourself the hassle of having to buy new scrubs frequently. Wash out Betadine (povidone-iodine) or benzoic stains on your scrubs with rubbing alcohol. Pour hydrogen peroxide on any blood spots on your uniform, and let foam for a minute. Then wash with soap and cold water. You may want to keep an extra pair of scrubs in your locker or car.
- Learn how to talk respectfully to others by reading up on how to engage effectively in crucial conversations.
- Enjoy your work and have a sense of humor, even if it seems unreasonable. You will not survive without one. Laughter is often the best medicine.
- Avoid gossip and be mindful about work-related posts on social media. Have you ever heard the phrase "nothing about me without me"? If someone is not present, then you should not be speaking about them. If you have an issue or question, resolve it by speaking directly to the person involved. We are all on the same team. We need to build each other up, not tear each other down. It is okay to seek advice on how to deal with certain situations; find a trustworthy mentor.
- Increase your ED knowledge. Join the Emergency Nurses Association, sign up for ED-related courses, and study from a certified emergency nurse (CEN) review book. Increasing your knowledge base is key for better patient care.
- Maintain liability insurance on yourself. It is inexpensive and almost everyone who works in the ED, at some point, gets sued. Liability insurance is a simple way to protect yourself.

- Document, document, document! How was the patient when he or she came in? Document airway, breathing, circulation, and neurological assessment findings. Develop good assessment skills early on, and know that patients do not always present according to the textbook. Chart on your nonurgent patient about once every hour; on a critical patient, as frequent as every 5 to 10 minutes. Chart when you assumed care of the patient. Document how the patient was when he or she left the ED (e.g., ambulatory, stable, age appropriate, alert) and reassess airway, breathing, and circulation (ABCs).

Fast Facts in a Nutshell

- Maintain liability insurance on yourself.
- Document, document, document!

SUMMARY

Emergency nursing is not for everyone. It can be indescribably hard at times, and everyone experiences a bad day here and there. But if you practice these simple stress-relieving techniques, you will be able to survive whatever the ED throws at you. If you can make it through the tough times, you will survive long enough to find out just how rewarding ED nursing can be. After all, isn't that why you chose this profession in the first place?

2

Acid–Base Imbalances

The body requires a delicate balance of acids and bases to maintain natural homeostasis. Many life-threatening illnesses affect the acid–base balance. Therefore, recognizing any acid–base imbalance is crucial to saving someone's life. As a nurse in the emergency department (ED), you will come across acid–base imbalances daily. Many new and experienced nurses find acid–base balance difficult to understand. After reviewing this chapter and learning the three simple steps provided, you will find it much easier to remember how to interpret test results. **Understanding the pathophysiology and reviewing many laboratory results are key to better understanding acid–base imbalances.**

During this part of your orientation, locate and become familiar with:

- Arterial blood gas procedures and results
- Diabetic ketoacidosis protocols
- Intubation equipment
- Medications to know: Insulin, sodium bicarbonate, potassium, and dextrose

PATHOPHYSIOLOGY

Acid–base balance is controlled by two organ systems.

Respiratory System

You breathe in oxygen (O_2) and breathe out carbon dioxide (CO_2). In the bloodstream CO_2 mixes with water (H_2O) to make **carbonic acid** (H_2CO_3).

Renal System

H_2CO_3 dissociates into a base, **bicarbonate** (HCO_3^-), and an acid (H^+), which is excreted or conserved by the kidneys. Normal pH of plasma contains a ratio of 20 bicarbonates to 1 carbonic acid.

Recognizing an Imbalance

An easy way to remember whether your patient has a respiratory or metabolic imbalance, as shown in Table 2.1, is this simple mnemonic.

For pH/bicarbonate directions in acidosis versus alkalosis, remember **ROME:**

Respiratory is **O**pposite (pH and CO_2), **M**etabolic is **E**qual (pH and HCO_3^-)

The arrows in Table 2.1 for respiratory pH and partial pressure of arterial carbon dioxide ($PaCO_2$) are in opposite directions from each other, and the arrows for metabolic pH and bicarbonate point in the same direction.

Fast Facts in a Nutshell

Acid–base balance is controlled by the respiratory and renal systems.

Table 2.1

Determining Acid–Base Imbalances			
Respiratory acidosis	pH↓	$PaCO_2$↑	HCO_3^- normal
Respiratory alkalosis	pH↑	$PaCO_2$↓	HCO_3^- normal
Metabolic acidosis	pH↓	$PaCO_2$ normal	HCO_3^-↓
Metabolic alkalosis	pH↑	$PaCO_2$ normal	HCO_3^-↑

Normal pH = 7.35–7.45; normal $PaCO_2$ = 35–45; normal HCO_3^- = 22–26.

HCO_3^-, bicarbonate; $PaCO_2$, partial pressure of carbon dioxide.

DIAGNOSES

Every acid–base imbalance is described using three words, such as uncompensated respiratory acidosis. To determine which imbalance your patient has, follow these three simple steps. Table 2.1 provides a visual guide of these steps.

- Look at the pH. If it is normal (7.35–7.45), it is *compensated.* If it is out of range, it is *uncompensated.*
- A pH less than 7.35 is *acidosis.* A pH greater than 7.45 is *alkalosis.*
- Look at $PaCO_2$ and HCO_3^-. Abnormal $PaCO_2$ = *respiratory.* Abnormal HCO_3^- = *metabolic.* If both are abnormal, it is both *respiratory* and *metabolic.*

Respiratory Acidosis

In respiratory acidosis, pH is less than 7.35 because of inadequate ventilations. Poor ventilation causes poor oxygenation and one to retain CO_2. That means O_2 cannot get in, and CO_2 cannot get out. CO_2 builds up and mixes with H_2O, resulting in H_2CO_3 lowering pH. HCO_3^- is normal. This patient is at risk for hypoxia.

- *Causes:* Upper airway obstruction; pulmonary edema; hypoventilation; head trauma; chest trauma; pneumonia; chronic obstructive pulmonary disease (COPD); narcotic overdose; and muscle weakness.
- *Signs and symptoms:* Tachycardia; headache; decreased pulse oximetry reading; confusion; weakness; coma; hyperkalemia; cyanosis; bradypnea; paralysis; and respiratory arrest.
- *Interventions:* Administer O_2; give nebulized breathing treatments; treat underlying condition; prepare for intubation; provide mechanical ventilation; measure pulse O_2; monitor cardiac rhythm; and obtain an intravenous access.

Notes: _____

Question: What supplies are needed to intubate a patient?
Answer: *High-flow O_2, suction, ambu bag, appropriate size endotracheal tube, 10-mL syringe of air, stylet, appropriate blades (Miller/Macintosh) with working handle, CO_2 detector, tape or endotracheal tube securing device, and stethoscope to check placement.*

Respiratory Alkalosis

In respiratory alkalosis, pH is greater than 7.45. When a person hyperventilates, he or she expels all of his or her CO_2. There is no CO_2 left to mix with H_2O to make H_2CO_3. No acid = alkalosis. HCO_3^- is normal.

- *Causes:* Hyperventilation; pain; anxiety; pulmonary embolus; hypoxia; high altitude; drug toxicity (early salicylate adult overdose); third-trimester pregnancy; and fever.
- *Signs and symptoms:* Tetany or seizures from hypocalcemia; diaphoresis; tingling of extremities; dizziness; altered mental status; anxiety; dyspnea; paresthesias; palpitations; tachycardia; and hyperventilation.
- *Interventions:* Encourage slow deep breathing; correct underlying condition; provide fluids intravenously; and correct hyperventilation with nonrebreather mask *without* O_2.
  - Hyperventilation treatment: Put O_2 nonrebreather mask over the patient's face and leave turned off. (It works like a paper bag.)

Notes: _____

Metabolic Acidosis

In metabolic acidosis, pH is less than 7.35 due to a decrease in HCO_3^- or increase in H^+ ion. $PaCO_2$ is normal. The kidneys compensate by excreting excess H^+ ions.

- *Causes:* Diabetic ketoacidosis; renal disease; starvation; shock or sepsis; and loss of bicarbonate in severe diarrhea.
- *Signs and symptoms:* Altered mental state; hypotension; abdominal pain; nausea, vomiting, and diarrhea; Kussmaul respirations; hyperventilation as a compensatory mechanism; tingling and

numbness; hyperkalemia; peaked T waves; flushed, warm skin; headache; bradycardia; and muscle weakness.

■ *Interventions:* Provide fluids intravenously (lactated ringer's); treatment may include intravenous sodium bicarbonate, intravenous dextrose, and intravenous regular insulin (to put potassium back in cells); assist ventilations; monitor cardiac rhythm; and perform basic metabolic panel (BMP).

Metabolic Alkalosis

In metabolic alkalosis, the pH is greater than 7.45 due to elevated HCO_3^- or decreased H^+. $PaCO_2$ is normal.

■ *Causes:* Loss of stomach acid associated with vomiting; ingesting too many alkali substances (antacids, milk of magnesia, or baking soda); diuretics; hypokalemia; and Cushing's syndrome.
■ *Signs and symptoms:* Hypocalcemia (tetany, twitching, irritability, shaking, and seizures); confusion; nausea, vomiting, and diarrhea; coma; decreased ST segment; bradypnea; hypokalemia (muscle weakness and loss of reflexes); and polyuria.
■ *Interventions:* Anticipate orders to prevent vomiting with antiemetics, avoid gastric suctioning, administer normal saline intravenously, perform BMP, provide potassium supplements for hypokalemia, and monitor cardiac performance and respirations.

Notes: _____

Question: Before your patient has an arterial blood gas drawn, what test should be performed?
Answer: *Allen's test.*

SUMMARY

Although acid–base imbalances can be challenging to understand, they are critical to maintaining natural homeostasis. An ED nurse comes across acid–base imbalances on a daily basis. Learn the steps provided in this chapter so you will be able to accurately interpret test results.

3

Cardiovascular Emergencies

In the emergency department (ED), cardiovascular diseases are an everyday life-threatening occurrence. However, **with proper assessment and fast treatment, cardiac diseases are resolved every day in EDs** across the country. After studying this chapter, you will have a basic understanding of cardiovascular assessments and treatments. This chapter does not replace electrocardiogram courses or the advanced cardiovascular life support certification required to work in the ED. **Many nurses find keeping an advanced cardiovascular life support handbook for study is very helpful.**

During this part of your orientation, locate and become familiar with:

- Electrocardiograms and supplies
- Advanced cardiovascular life support and electrocardiogram courses available to you
- Cardiac monitors, defibrillators, and pacers
- Crash carts
- Pacer magnets
- Medications to know: Aspirin, morphine, nitroglycerin, atropine, adenosine, digoxin, furosemide, calcium channel blockers, beta-blockers, amiodarone, lidocaine, epinephrine, vasopressin, heparin, warfarin, dopamine, nicardipine hydrochloride, and norepinephrine

DIAGNOSES

Congestive Heart Failure

In congestive heart failure, the heart fails to pump blood effectively. It can be acute or chronic. As a result, blood backs up. It can back up to the body (right-sided congestive heart failure) or the lungs (left-sided congestive heart failure).

- *Causes:* Other illnesses can, over time, lead to congestive heart failure. These include hypertension; arrhythmias; diabetes; coronary artery disease; valvular stenosis; cardiomyopathy; emphysema; obesity; pulmonary embolism; anemia; and thyroid disease.
- *Signs and symptoms:*
  - *Right sided:* Pitting pedal edema; hepatojugular reflux; liver enlargement; nocturia; and jugular vein distention.
  - *Left sided:* Usually develops first; crackles; shortness of breath; pulmonary edema (rales); tachypnea; left ventricular hypertrophy; tachycardia; and ventricular gallop.
- *Interventions:* Administer oxygen; establish intravenous (IV) access; monitor cardiac performance; and administer medications as ordered (e.g., furosemide, morphine, and nitroglycerin).
  - Monitor intake and output. Provide condom catheter, urinal, bedside commode, or bedpan for frequent urination after furosemide administration.

Notes: _____

Question: Which patient position is best to hear S3 (ventricular gallop) and S4 (atrial gallop)?
Answer: *Left lateral.*

Acute Myocardial Infarction

Acute myocardial infarction is the result of a clogged coronary artery supplying blood to the heart muscle. The patient's history often reveals hypertension, coronary artery disease, high cholesterol, and smoking (see Figure 3.1).

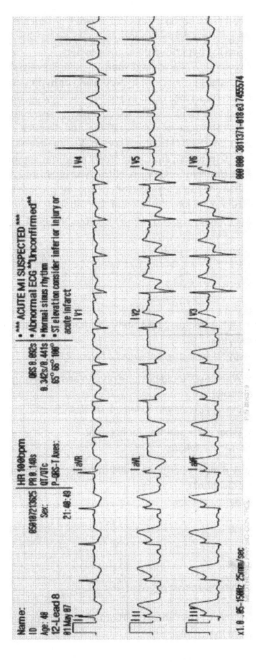

Figure 3.1 Suspected acute myocardial infarction.

Chapter 3 Cardiovascular Emergencies

- *Causes:* Blood clots; coronary arterial spasm from cocaine use. Contributing factors: hypertension; coronary artery disease; smoking; obesity; hyperlipidemia; and genetics.
- *Signs and symptoms:* Nausea and vomiting; diaphoresis; shortness of breath; fatigue; anxiety; hypertension or hypotension; and chest pain (described often as pressure, squeezing, tightness, or vague) that may radiate to the left shoulder or jaw. Females may present with vague weakness, fatigue, and dyspnea.
- *Interventions: MOVE!!* (**M**onitor, **O**xygen, **V**enous access, and **E**KG within 10 minutes); anticipate orders to administer medications **MONA** (**M**orphine, **O**xygen, **N**itroglycerin SL, and **A**spirin), obtain cardiac enzymes, arrange for chest x-ray, prepare for possible cardiac cath lab admission or thrombolytic or anticoagulant (heparin) therapy, and reassess/monitor chest pain.

Notes: _____

Question: What factors absolutely contraindicate the use of thrombolytics?
Answer: *Active bleeding, recent surgery, or recent trauma.*

Question: What test should be done prior to administering heparin or thrombolytics?
Answer: *Stool hemoccult and coagulant studies.*

Question: What is the antidote for heparin?
Answer: *Protamine sulfate.*

Question: A patient allergic to shellfish might also be allergic to what medication?
Answer: *Protamine sulfate.*

Arterial Occlusion

Arterial occlusion means a clogged artery.

- *Causes:* Coronary artery disease; atherosclerosis; hypertension; smoking; and hyperlipidemia.

- *Signs and symptoms:* Cool/pale extremities and weak pulse to the affected extremity.
- *Interventions:* Maintain extremity in dependent position; assess pulses through Doppler ultrasound; and prepare for possible surgery.

Notes: _____

Endocarditis

Endocarditis is an infection of the inner lining of the heart and/or the heart valves.

- *Causes:* Endocarditis occurs when a person with faulty heart valves contracts a common bacterial infection. For example, a bacterial infection in the skin can travel through the blood and attach to the faulty heart valve, resulting in endocarditis.
- *Signs and symptoms:* Chills; fever; splinter hemorrhaging of the nail beds; chest pain; and systolic murmur.
- *Interventions:* Anticipate orders to obtain multiple blood cultures from multiple sites, administer antibiotics intravenously, and do a complete blood count.

Notes: _____

Aortic Injuries

Aortic injuries may occur anywhere on the ascending aorta, aortic arch, descending thoracic aorta, or abdominal aorta. The injuries can result in aneurysm, tear, or rupture. Without immediate surgery the patient can bleed to death rapidly. So it is critical for the nurse to identify an aortic injury early.

- *Causes:* A history of aortic injuries may reveal hypertension; coronary artery disease; congestive heart failure; or a recent chest/abdominal trauma.
- *Signs and symptoms* (may vary depending on location): Hypotension; loss of consciousness; hypertension in upper extremities; stronger pulse in arms than in legs; tearing chest pain that radiates to the back; tearing abdominal pain; chest wall ecchymosis; and paraplegia.

■ *Interventions:* Get patient on a stretcher; obtain vital signs; check blood pressure in all extremities; notify provider of patient signs and symptoms immediately; prepare for immediate surgery; start two large-bore IV lines; monitor cardiac performance; provide oxygen; perform electrocardiogram; and measure pulse oximetry.

Notes: _____

Question: Which type of trauma most commonly causes a descending thoracic aortic laceration?
Answer: *Deceleration trauma that causes shearing.*

Symptomatic Bradycardia

In symptomatic bradycardia, heart rate is less than 60 beats per minute resulting in inadequate blood circulation. The patient is symptomatic, displaying signs of poor cardiac perfusion (see Figure 3.2).

■ *Causes:* The cause is not always known, but underlying conditions such as coronary artery disease, heart disease, second- or third-degree heart blocks, hypertension, thyroid disease, and lung disease can contribute to bradycardia.

■ *Signs and symptoms:* Heart rate lower than 60 beats per minute; patient looks and feels unwell (e.g., altered loss of consciousness, chest pain, diaphoretic, and pale).

■ *Interventions:* Assess airway, breathing, and circulation (ABCs); provide oxygen; check vital signs; measure pulse oxygen; perform electrocardiogram; monitor cardiac performance; anticipate orders to intravenously push 0.5 to 1.0 mg of atropine at 3- to 5-minute intervals, establish transcutaneous pacing, administer medications (dopamine or epinephrine), and prepare for transcutaneous (external) or internal pacer.

Notes: _____

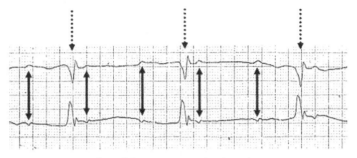

Figure 3.2 Symptomatic bradycardia.

Supraventricular Tachycardia

In supraventricular tachycardia, the heart rate is regular but it beats at more than 150 beats per minute. Supraventricular tachycardia can be divided into symptomatic/unstable (patient looks unwell) or asymptomatic/stable (patient looks fine; see Figure 3.3).

- *Causes:* The cause is not always known. However, some habits and conditions can contribute to it, such as stress, caffeine, smoking, cocaine use, alcohol use, thyroid disease, heart failure, pulmonary embolism, chronic obstructive pulmonary disease, and pneumonia. Some medications for asthma, cold medications, and digoxin can also contribute to supraventricular tachycardia.
- *Signs and symptoms:* Palpitations; chest pain; diaphoresis; anxiety; and pulse rate greater than 150 beats per minute.
- *Interventions:*
  - *If patient is symptomatic and unstable,* anticipate order to prepare for immediate synchronized cardioversion 50 to 100 J biphasic.
  - *If patient is asymptomatic and stable,* anticipate orders to attempt vasovagal maneuvers, monitor cardiac performance, open large-bore IV line, provide oxygen, check vital signs, measure pulse oxygen, perform electrocardiogram, administer adenosine rapidly by IV push, and slow down atrioventricular (AV) conduction with beta-blockers/calcium channel blockers/digoxin or amiodarone.
    - Give patient a coffee straw and ask him or her to blow through it to assist vagal maneuvers.

Notes: _____

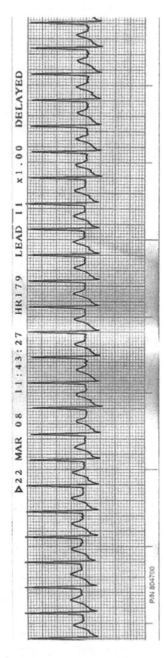

▷22 MAR 08   11:43:27   HR179   LEAD II   x1.00   DELAYED

P/N 804700

Figure 3.3 Supraventricular tachycardia.

Ventricular Fibrillation or Pulseless Ventricular Tachycardia

Ventricular fibrillation (VF) and pulseless ventricular tachycardia (VT) are both irregular rapid rhythms in which there is no pulse (see Figure 3.4 and Table 3.1).

- *Causes:* Poor cardiac perfusion due to coronary artery disease; shock; hypokalemia; myocardial infarct; or electrocution.
- *Signs and symptoms:* Decreased level of consciousness; no pulse; VF or VT on cardiac monitor.
- *Interventions:* Assess for a pulse within 10 seconds; if no pulse present, call for help while initiating cardiopulmonary resuscitation (CPR) starting with chest compressions; do not interrupt chest compressions while applying cardiac monitor/ defibrillation pads. Pulseless VT or VF are shockable rhythms. Be sure you know how to set your machine to defibrillation mode and always make sure your team is all clear before pressing the shock button. Anticipate orders to administer early defibrillation, epinephrine, and amiodarone or lidocaine per advanced cardiovascular life support protocols. Just remember DEAL: Defibrillation, Epinephrine, and Amiodarone or Lidocaine.

Notes: _____

Table 3.1

Pulseless Ventricular Tachycardia or Ventricular Fibrillation Treatment

1. Shock at 120–200 J biphasic
   - CPR 30/2 for five cycles or 2 min
   - Epinephrine 1 mg IV/IO during CPR every 3–5 min
2. Shock at 200 J biphasic if still pulseless VT or VF after 2 min CPR
   - CPR 30/2 for five cycles or 2 min
   - Amiodarone 300 mg, 150 mg second dose or lidocaine during CPR
3. Shock at 200 J biphasic if still pulseless VT or VF after 2 min CPR
   - CPR 30/2 for five cycles or 2 min
   - Consider magnesium 1–2 g IV/IO for torsades de pointes

CPR, cardiopulmonary resuscitation; IO, intraosseous; IV, intravenous; VF, ventricular fibrillation; VT, ventricular tachycardia.

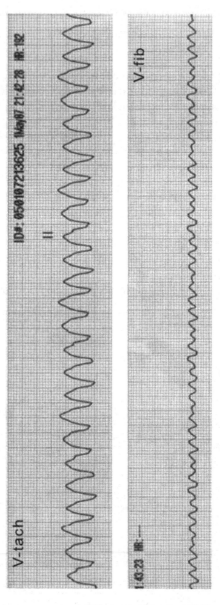

Figure 3.4 Ventricular fibrillation.

Question: If none of the above interventions work, what are some other causes of VF?

Answer: *Hypothermia, hypoxia, hypoglycemia, overdose, cardiac tamponade, tension pneumothorax, trauma, acidosis, hypovolemia, and electrolyte imbalances.*

Question: You see VF on the monitor, but your patient is asymptomatic, sitting up, and talking to you. What is your first intervention?

Answer: *Check for a pulse. You cannot believe everything you see on a monitor; it could be artifact.*

Question: What is the maximum number of times one can safely defibrillate a patient?

Answer: *There is no limit.*

Question: Why do we defibrillate?

Answer: *To temporarily produce asystole. This may sound incorrect, but defibrillation actually depolarizes the heart, allowing the natural pacemakers of the heart to kick in.*

Question: What dose of lidocaine should be administered to patients with renal failure, liver failure, or patients who are elderly?

Answer: *Give half doses of lidocaine to patients with renal failure, patients with liver failure, or patients who are elderly.*

Pulseless Electrical Activity

Pulseless electrical activity occurs when a rhythm shows on the monitor, but the patient does not have a pulse. Again, you cannot always believe what you see on the monitor.

- *Causes:* Can be attributed to the five **H**s or five **T**s.
    - **H**ypovolemia, **H**ypoxia, **H**ydrogen ion (acidosis), **H**yper-/hypokalemia, or **H**ypothermia.
    - **T**oxin (drug overdose), **T**amponade/cardiac, **T**ension pneumothorax, **T**hrombosis, and **T**rauma.
- *Signs and symptoms:* Your patient has no pulse, but there is a rhythm on the monitor. Remember that just because there is

electrical activity in the heart does not mean the heart is actually pumping.

- *Interventions:* Check for a pulse; if no pulse, perform CPR starting with chest compressions; per order, insert an IV line, monitor oxygen, and administer epinephrine.

Notes: _____

Question: What is the effect of nitroprusside (Nipride) administered intravenously?
Answer: *It reduces afterload and increases cardiac output. It decreases myocardial oxygen demand without affecting the heart rate.*

Question: What type of electrocardiogram changes might you see in a patient with a potassium level of 7.8?
Answer: *Bradycardia, peaked T waves, and widened QRS complex.*

Question: What equation defines cardiac output?
Answer: *Heart rate × stroke volume.*

Question: What are the manifestations of digoxin toxicity?
Answer: *Blurred vision, halos, and arrhythmias.*

Question: What is the treatment for digoxin toxicity?
Answer: *Glucagon, phenytoin (Dilantin), and digoxin immune fab (Digibind).*

Question: Name three vasopressors.
Answer: *Norepinephrine, dopamine, and metaraminol are vasopressors.*

Question: What is the antidote for warfarin (Coumadin)?
Answer: *Vitamin K.*

Fast Facts in a Nutshell

- Heparin affects partial thromboplastin time.
- Warfarin (Coumadin) affects prothrombin time.

SUMMARY

Although cardiovascular diseases threaten lives every day, they can often be resolved with quick treatment. An ED nurse needs to understand the basics of cardiovascular assessments and treatments and be certified in advanced cardiovascular life support.

Chapter 3 **Cardiovascular Emergencies**

4

Dental, Ear, Nose, and Throat Emergencies

Dental, ear, nose, and throat emergencies are daily occurrences in the emergency department (ED). **Most of the time, they are not life-threatening.** From foreign objects to trauma or infection, this chapter takes you through the most common dental, ear, nose, and throat emergencies you will face. For each emergency, you will learn causes, manifestations, and interventions.

During this part of your orientation, locate and become familiar with:

- Dental repair kit and its contents
- Alligator forceps
- Ear wicks
- Eardrops for infection and cerumen impaction
- Ear irrigation supplies and ear curettes
- Headlamp and otoscope
- Nasal packing supplies

DIAGNOSES

Dental Abscess

A dental abscess is a pocket of infection and/or pus located in the gums near the base of a tooth.

- *Causes:*
  - *Periodontal abscess:* An infection of the soft tissue related to periodontitis (gum disease) or foreign object.
  - *Periapical abscess:* An infection of the supporting bone around the root structure caused by damage to the pulp (nerve and blood supply) of the tooth.
- *Signs and symptoms:* Manifestation may vary depending on location, but usually includes pain, swelling, toothache, tenderness, fever, and foul breath. Infection may be localized but may also spread into areas of the face and neck. Pain may radiate to neck, jaw, and ear.
- *Interventions:* Assess and treat any airway obstructions first. Anticipate orders to set up oral anesthetics and incision and drainage tray or supplies, and administer any intravenous fluids, pain medication, and antibiotics as ordered. Anticipate diagnostic study orders such as complete blood count, arterial blood gas, erythrocyte sedimentation rate, wound cultures of the abscess, and computed tomography (CT) or soft tissue x-ray of the head and neck.

Fractured Tooth

A tooth fracture is a broken or chipped tooth. This commonly occurs to the "two front teeth" or anterior maxillary teeth as a result of trauma.

- *Causes:* Oral, facial, or head trauma.
- *Signs and symptoms:* Vary according to type and location of trauma and may include broken or chipped tooth, bleeding at site of injury, pain, swelling, and/or embedded tooth fragments.
- *Interventions:* If facial trauma is present, stabilize any airway, breathing, or circulation concerns first. Consider tooth aspiration. Then place warm moist cotton over the exposed tooth fracture and cover with dry gauze. Administer oral analgesics and tetanus vaccine as ordered. Consider abuse if caregiver history does not match that of the patient. Referral to a dentist within 24 to 48 hours of injury is critical for proper tooth repair. Set up emergency dental repair kit for provider administration.

Fast Facts in a Nutshell

An emergency dental repair kit, box, or supplies for provider administration may include zinc oxide, nerve-blocking agent, calcium hydroxide, intermediate restorative material (IMR), dental foil, dental cement, and/or dry socket paste.

Odontalgia

"Odontalgia" is a big fancy word for dental caries or "cavities." Commonly, patients show up to the emergency department for the severe pain associated with odontalgia.

- *Causes:* Poor oral hygiene and a diet high in sugar.
- *Signs and symptoms:* Pain; gray or blackened area noted on affected tooth; toothache; and neck or facial swelling.
- *Interventions:* May include administration of topical anesthetics, nerve blocks, narcotic analgesics, IMR, and antibiotics. However, these treatments do not cure odontalgia; they simply buy the patient some time until he or she sees the dentist. Stress importance of good oral hygiene and need for following up with dentist during discharge instructions.

Tooth Avulsion

Tooth avulsion occurs when the whole tooth is removed from its socket. This is a time-sensitive emergency. The best chance of saving the tooth is reimplantation *within 30 minutes.*

- *Causes:* Commonly head, facial, or oral trauma of some sort.
- *Signs and symptoms:* Missing tooth; bleeding; pain; and swelling. Hopefully your patient found the missing tooth and brought it in to the ED with him or her.
- *Interventions:* If facial trauma is present, stabilize any airway, breathing, or circulation concerns first. Consider tooth aspiration. Tooth and socket should be gently cleansed with tap water and any debris removed. Attempt should be made to place the cleansed tooth back in its socket. If tooth will not stay in socket, tooth should be placed in a liquid medium such as milk or saliva.

Administer oral analgesics and tetanus vaccine as ordered. Referral to a dentist within 24 to 48 hours of injury is critical for proper tooth repair. Set up dental repair kit, box, or supplies for provider administration as ordered. Discharge teaching should include the use of helmets and mouth guards when playing sports.

Question: Which liquid media are appropriate for avulsed teeth?
Answer: *Saliva, milk, or Hank's solution (an over-the-counter product).*

Ludwig's Angina

Ludwig's angina occurs when a preexisting dental infection or cellulitis spreads into the sublingual, submandibular, and/or submental mandibular spaces.

- *Causes:* The spreading of a preexisting dental infection.
- *Signs and symptoms:* Anterior or lateral neck swelling; tongue swelling; pain; drooling; dysphagia; fever; and chills.
- *Interventions:* The swelling related to this particular type of infection places your patient at high risk for airway obstruction. Assess and maintain patent airway, breathing, and circulation. Anticipate orders to administer oxygen, intravenous fluids, pain medication, and antibiotics; attach pulse oximeter and cardiac monitor; set up for incision and drainage; and/or prepare for operating room (OR) admission. Diagnostic tests may include arterial blood gas, complete blood count, erythrocyte sedimentation rate, culture of oral infected wound or drainage, and head and neck soft tissue x-rays or CT.

Foreign Objects

You name it, it can be found in an ear or a nostril. It commonly occurs with curious young children and toddlers, but occasionally with adult patients. Hopefully, the object will be detected before infection occurs. Getting it out of the uncooperative 3-year-old patient is the real trick!

- *Causes:* Foreign object in the ear, such as nuts, bolts, raisins, peas, beads, bugs, and cotton.

- *Signs and symptoms:* Visible foreign object; purulent or bloody discharge; discomfort or pain; swelling; redness; foul odor; and foreign body sensation.
- *Interventions:*
  - Remove the foreign body with suction, irrigation, alligator forceps, or ear curette. Provide ear antibiotics or nasal decongestants as ordered. Instruct the patient not to put anything smaller than an elbow in his or her ears or nose!
  - Sometimes nasal foreign bodies can be dislodged simply by closing off the unaffected nostril and asking the patient to blow forcefully out of the affected nostril.
  - If unable to remove foreign body, provider may refer patient to ear, nose, and throat specialist.

Notes: _____

Fast Facts in a Nutshell

There are many ways to flush an ear, but this seems to work the best for wax removal.

- First, gather lukewarm water with a splash of peroxide mixed in a small basin and a 20-mL syringe with plastic needle-less short tip. You can also cut off the end of an intravenous catheter.
- Lay the patient on his or her side with affected ear up. Fill the ear canal with warm water and peroxide solution and let soak for 10 minutes. Then sit patient up with basin under ear to catch fluids. Now that the wax is softened, irrigate ear canal using syringe and rest of water solution. If a brown scaly pebble comes out, this is the wax impaction; you got it!

Acute Otitis Externa (Swimmer's Ear)

Acute otitis externa is a bacterial or fungal infection of the outer ear.

- *Causes:* Outer ear infections commonly occur because of frequent swimming or foreign objects in the ear. Bacteria or fungus enters with the water or the foreign object, thereby causing an infection.
- *Signs and symptoms:* Outer ear pain; itchy, impaired hearing; ear discharge; fever; erythema; and swelling of the outer ear.

- *Interventions:* Give topical eardrop solution/antibiotics as ordered; provide ear wick; and use warm compresses. Instruct the patient not to swim until the infection is resolved (7–10 days).

Notes: _____

Fast Facts in a Nutshell

- When examining the ear in an adult, pull *up* and back; in a child under 3 years of age, pull the ear *down* and back.

Acute Otitis Media

Acute otitis media is a middle-ear bacterial or viral infection. It is more common in children because of their short, narrow Eustachian tubes. An infant or toddler with otitis media may appear irritable, cry, pull at ears, and have a poor appetite, nausea, vomiting, or diarrhea.

- *Causes:* Middle-ear infections usually start as a sinus infection.
- *Signs and symptoms:* Recent upper respiratory infection; earache; impaired hearing; red or dull gray bulging tympanic membrane; and fever.
- *Interventions:* Administer and evaluate effectiveness of antipyretics, antibiotics, and pain medication as ordered.

Notes: _____

Ruptured Tympanic Membrane

This is a tear or rupture of the tympanic membrane (eardrum).

- *Causes:* Tears may be the result of infection or trauma from a foreign object (Q-tip, bobby pin) or other forces (e.g., explosions, skull fractures, burns).
- *Signs and symptoms:* Ear pain; discharge; impaired hearing; vertigo; nausea, vomiting, and fever.
- *Interventions:* With most small perforations, the eardrum grows back on its own, similar to the way a fingernail grows back. Anticipate orders to administer oral antibiotics, prepare for

surgery in large perforations; instruct patient not to blow nose or get ears wet, and provide follow-up with an ear, nose, and throat specialist.

Notes: _____

Ménière's Disease

Ménière's disease is an inner-ear disorder affecting adults between 40 and 50 years of age.

- *Causes:* Its cause is unknown. Symptoms usually occur suddenly and can last from a few minutes to a few hours.
- *Signs and symptoms:* Vertigo; dizziness; nausea and vomiting; tinnitus; impaired hearing; diaphoresis; headache; and blurred vision.
- *Interventions:* Bring side rails up (fall precautions) and put the bed in the low-locked position; speak slowly and clearly; administer diazepam (intravenously) for rapid relief and antiemetics as ordered; require bed rest and a quiet environment; and provide diet instructions (low sodium, no caffeine, and no nicotine).

Notes: _____

Allergic Rhinitis (Hay Fever)

Rhinitis is a nasal mucous membrane inflammation.

- *Causes:* Allergic response to pollen, dust, or other allergens. It may be acute (seasonal) or chronic (perennial).
- *Signs and symptoms:* Watery nasal drainage; nasal congestion; sneezing; cough; and sore throat. Infants may present with difficulty breathing or poor feeding.
- *Interventions:* Administer medications as ordered (analgesics, antibiotics, decongestants, and antihistamines); increase fluid intake; and perform bulb syringe suction in infants.

Notes: _____

Epistaxis

Epistaxis is a nose bleed. There are two types: anterior bleeds and posterior bleeds.

Anterior bleeds are more common and easier to control.

- *Causes:* Trauma; cocaine use; disease; nose picking; or just dry air during winter months.
- *Signs and symptoms:* Bright red nasal bleeding.
- *Interventions:* Position patient sitting up and leaning forward; apply direct pressure to bridge of nose; apply ice; administer medications as ordered (pseudoephedrine); and prepare for cauterization or nasal packing.

Posterior bleeds are less common and more difficult to control.

- *Causes:* Usually associated with chronic medical problems, such as hypertension, blood dyscrasia, or tumor.
- *Signs and symptoms:* Nasal bleeding.
- *Interventions:* Apply direct pressure and ice for 10 minutes or more. Position the patient sitting up and leaning forward over a large basin. Establish large-bore intravenous access, if ordered; have suction and headlamp available; arrange for ear, nose, and throat consult as ordered; prepare for procedure (posterior nasal packing, nasal tampon, or cauterization); and monitor level of consciousness, vital signs, pulse oxygen, and bleeding. *Instruct patient not to blow nose.*

Notes: _____

Nasal Fracture

This is a fracture of the nasal bones.

- *Causes:* Direct trauma to the nose.
- *Signs and symptoms:* Nasal bleeding; nasal ecchymosis or edema; nasal airway obstruction; and deformity or tenderness over nasal bridge.
- *Interventions:* Control bleeding with direct pressure; apply ice; administer analgesics as ordered and evaluate effectiveness;

and arrange for nasal or facial x-ray. *Instruct patient not to blow nose.*

■ If nasal airway is not obstructed, no treatment is necessary.
■ If nasal airway is obstructed, patient will be referred to an ear, nose, and throat specialist for repair *1 week after swelling decreases.*

Notes: _____

Sinusitis

Sinusitis is a sinus inflammation.

■ *Causes:* Infection; allergies; chemical irritants; pressure changes; cocaine use; dental abscesses; or mechanical obstruction.
■ *Signs and symptoms:* Pain; purulent nasal drainage; and fever.
■ *Interventions:* Anticipate orders to administer medications and evaluate effectiveness (decongestants, antibiotic, and analgesic/ narcotic); and arrange for sinus films or CT scan.

Notes: _____

Pharyngitis/Tonsillitis

This is inflammation of the throat or tonsils.

■ *Causes:* Bacterial or viral infection.
■ *Signs and symptoms:* Sore throat; red swollen tonsils; white pus on tonsils; difficulty swallowing; fever; ear pain; foul breath; and swollen cervical lymph nodes.
■ *Interventions:* Arrange for strep or monospot test; administer antibiotic by mouth (PO) or injection (IM) as ordered; and monitor airway patency.
  ■ Soft tissue neck x-ray may be used to rule out *epiglottitis* or retropharyngeal abscess when patient demonstrates pain, drooling, "hot-potato voice," or difficulty in breathing.

Notes: _____

Peritonsillar Abscess

This is an abscess of the tonsil. It may be a respiratory emergency if the airway is obstructed.

- *Causes:* Commonly caused by streptococcus bacteria.
- *Signs and symptoms:* Sore throat; unilateral swollen tonsil; swollen cervical lymph nodes; dysphagia; fever; difficulty in opening mouth; swollen palate; laterally displaced uvula; drooling; and muffled or "hot-potato voice."
- *Interventions:* Prepare for incision and drainage of abscess with ear, nose, and throat consultant; administer antibiotics and pulse oxygen; and monitor airway.

Notes: _____

Question: What is the difference between tonsillitis and peritonsillar abscess?
Answer: *With tonsillitis, both tonsils are swollen. With peritonsillar abscess, one tonsil is swollen.*

SUMMARY

You should now have a basic understanding of the dental, ear, nose, and throat problems that are seen daily in the ED. Do not be afraid to take an otoscope and assess your patient's mouth, gums, and teeth, ears, nose, or throat. Most providers appreciate a good assessment, especially one that is well documented before and after treatment.

5

Disaster Response Emergencies

Working in the emergency department (ED) automatically makes you a first responder during a local disaster. Therefore, it is vital to know your role, communicate effectively, and locate equipment quickly. Disasters can be divided into two categories: natural and man-made. This chapter opens with the definitions, categories, and interventions for disasters. Many nurses may find remembering disaster instructions difficult because, quite simply, they are rarely used. Never fear. Just learn these three helpful mnemonics to remember what to do: **DISASTER, SALT,** and **IDMED.** Then, the chapter guides you through some of the most common radiological, chemical, and biological exposures. Again, you may find it challenging to remember information that is used so infrequently, so just keep this book and the Centers for Disease Control and Prevention (CDC) website handy. These two sources will provide all the information you need. To fully understand the material and ease your anxiety, be sure to practice an actual disaster drill in your facility during your orientation.

During this part of your orientation, locate and become familiar with:

- Your facility's disaster plans
- Your facility's disaster codes
- Decontamination equipment
- Fire alarms and extinguishers

(continued)

- Oxygen shut-off valves
- Evacuation plans and routes
- Contacts/whom to notify if a disaster occurs
- Where to sign up to participate in a disaster drill
- Disaster communication routes
- Personal protective equipment (PPE) for highly infectious diseases
- Hazmat suits
- Hospital disaster supplies

TYPES OF DISASTERS

A "disaster" is an event in which needs exceed resources. The types are indicated in Table 5.1.

Table 5.1

Types of Disasters	
Natural	**Man-made**
Hurricane	Explosion
Earthquake	Fire
Landslide	Firearms
Ice storm/blizzard	Stampede
Fire	Structural collapse
Wildfire	Hazardous material
Flood	Power out
Tidal wave	Blocked communications
Tornado	Transportation event
Asteroid collision	■ Airway (Plane)
Avalanche	■ Railway (Train)
	■ Waterway (Boat)
Volcanic eruption	■ Roadway (Car)
	Weapons of mass destruction
	■ Biological
	■ Chemical
	■ Nuclear

INTERVENTIONS

To remember the proper interventions to follow in a disaster, remember the mnemonics DISASTER, SALT, and IDMED.

DISASTER

- **D**etect: What is the reason for the disaster. Are there mass casualties? Do our needs exceed our resources?
- **I**ncident command: People trained to manage, coordinate, and organize the disaster operation. Do we need them and, if so, where?
- **S**afe and secure scene: Is it safe? Always protect yourself and team members first, then the public, patients, and environment. Use PPE, such as gown, gloves, and mask.
- **A**ssess hazards: What are other potential hazards (e.g., downed power lines, blood, smoke, leaking gas line, bad weather)?
- **S**upport: What people and supplies are needed? Do we need hazmat team, fire and rescue team, law enforcement, vehicles, water?
- **T**riage and treatment: Do we need triage? How much treatment is required? Follow your facility's disaster triage plan. If your facility does not have one, you can locate one online through the Federal Emergency Management Agency. See SALT and IDMED mnemonics in the following.
- **E**vacuate: Can the victims be transported to a safe location and, if so, how?
- **R**ecovery: What are some recovery issues?

SALT

- **S**ort or prioritize patients into one of three categories based on movement by calling out to the victims:
  - "Those who can walk, come to this location." These are Priority 3: able to walk.
  - "Those who can hear my voice, wave your hand." These are Priority 2: able to wave with purposeful movement.
  - "Those who do not respond." These are Priority 1: still with obvious threats to life.
- **A**ssess the victims who cannot walk or move, as they are more urgent and need assistance.
- **L**imited life-saving interventions: If indicated, perform the following:
  - Open the airway through repositioning.

- ▪ Perform needle chest decompression.
- ▪ Control major hemorrhage with direct pressure or tourniquet.
- ▪ Administer autoinjector antidotes.
- ■ Triage and transport: Triage or sort patients using the IDMED mnemonic. Transport the immediate first, then delayed, minimal, expectant, and dead.

IDMED

- ■ **I**mmediate, Emergent, or Red acuity: These victims have an alteration in airway, breathing, and circulation (ABCs) or threat to loss of life or limb.
- ■ **D**elayed, Urgent, or Yellow acuity: These victims need medical attention, but they are not at risk of rapidly deteriorating.
- ■ **M**inimal, Nonurgent, or Green acuity: These victims have stable vital signs and minor wounds.
- ■ **E**xpectant or Blue acuity: These victims have little or no chance of survival with current resources.
- ■ **D**ead: These victims have no pulse or respirations.

Send immediate victims to hospital/operating room/intensive care unit first.

Fast Facts in a Nutshell

To remember the proper interventions to follow in a disaster, remember the mnemonics **DISASTER, SALT,** and **IDMED**.

RADIATION, CHEMICAL, AND BIOLOGICAL EXPOSURES

Emergency medical personnel should always wear PPE, remove contaminated clothing, clean objects in 1% bleach solution, wash patient in proper decontamination showering systems, and report to infection control at the CDC at https://wwwn.cdc.gov/dcs/ContactUs/Form (1-800-CDC-INFO).

Abrin or Ricin

Abrin or ricin toxicity results from biological exposure to processed castor beans.

- *Causes:* Contact with poison released from processed castor beans, such as might occur at a castor bean plant. The poison inactivates type II ribosomes in the body.
- *Signs and symptoms:* Within a few days, metabolic acidosis; hepatitis; renal failure; and hematuria.
    - *If poison is inhaled:* Within 4 to 8 hours, the patient will experience distress, fever, cough, shortness of breath, pulmonary edema, lung necrosis, and shock.
    - *If poison is ingested:* Nausea, vomiting, and diarrhea; rectal bleeding; hypotension; gastrointestinal necrosis; and hepatitis.
- *Interventions:* Decontaminate the patient with proper equipment; use standard precautions; administer fluids intravenously per order; and avoid exposure to contaminated substances. There is no antidote; treat the symptoms. Give charcoal, if ingestion is recent.

Notes: _____

Anthrax

Anthrax is a spore-forming gram-positive bacteria (*Bacillus anthracis*).

- *Causes:* Contaminated soil, animals, and animal products. The bacteria enter the body through inhalation, skin, or ingestion.
- *Signs and symptoms:*
    - *If spore is inhaled:* Within 2 to 40+ days, flu-like symptoms, including weakness; cough; congestion; sore throat; fever; shortness of breath; respiratory distress; and shock.
    - *If spore enters subcutaneously:* Within a week, an itchy vesicle turns into an ulcer and then a black scab, possibly with fever (see Figure 5.1).
    - *If spore is ingested:* Within a week, nausea, vomiting, and diarrhea; rectal bleeding; and fever.
- *Interventions:* Anticipate orders to obtain blood cultures, arrange for chest x-ray and CT scan, give antibiotics such as ciprofloxacin, and use standard precautions.

Notes: _____

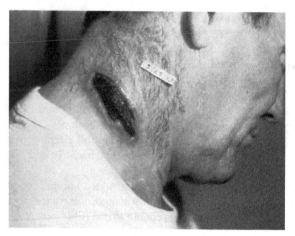

Figure 5.1 Subcutaneous anthrax.

Fast Facts in a Nutshell

The inhaled form of anthrax has a very high fatality rate.

Botulism

Botulism is a paralyzing toxin produced by the bacteria *Clostridium botulinum*.

- *Causes:* Contaminated food; infected wounds; and spore consumption (e.g., honey) by infants.
- *Signs and symptoms:* Within 4 days, patient has multiple cranial nerve palsies. The patient is also afebrile with bilateral facial droop; dysphonia; blurred vision; normal mental status; dry mouth; dysphagia; dysarthria; and bilateral descending skeletal muscle paralysis. Respiratory failure occurs in 24 hours or less.
- *Interventions:* Standard precautions; assess neurological status; monitor cardiac performance; measure pulse oxygen; collect gastric or stool samples; use ventilator if patient is experiencing respiratory failure; and give antitoxin available through state health departments and the CDC as ordered.

Notes: _____

Question: An infant is brought into the ED for facial droop, muscle weakness, and shallow respirations. Botulism is suspected. What does this patient need from the CDC?
Answer: *Antitoxin.*

Blister Agent (Mustard Gas)

A blister agent is an alkaline agent with a mustard, onion, or garlic odor.

- *Causes:* The gas is an agent used in chemical warfare that results in blisters and burns.
- *Signs and symptoms:* Within 12 hours, the patient experiences second-degree burns; skin redness with blisters; corneal abrasions; sore throat; nausea, vomiting, and diarrhea; cough; and difficulty in breathing.
- *Interventions:* Decontaminate patient; perform ABCs first; and treat symptoms, particularly chemical burns, with topical antibiotics as ordered. There is no antidote.

Notes: _____

Brucellosis

Brucellosis is a bacterial (*Brucella*) infection.

- *Causes:* Infected animals or animal products.
- *Signs and symptoms:* Within 4 weeks, the patient experiences fever; flu-like symptoms; sweating; headache; weakness; hepatitis; joint pain; arthritis; osteomyelitis; and endocarditis.
- *Interventions:* Use standard precautions; and anticipate orders to obtain blood cultures and give antibiotics (doxycycline and rifampin).

Notes: _____

Cyanide

Cyanide is a colorless chemical gas or crystal that binds with cellular mitochondria preventing adenosine triphosphate (ATP) production. It has a bitter almond odor. Example: "Jonestown Massacre" of 1978 where 909 Americans died by drinking cyanide poisoned punch or Kool-Aid.

- *Causes:* Gas or crystals found in manufacturing; certain foods; and cigarette smoke.
- *Signs and symptoms:* Bradypnea; dizziness; weakness; headache; nausea; vomiting; tachycardia or bradycardia; hypotension; loss of consciousness; and respiratory failure.
- *Interventions:* Decontaminate patient; assess and treat ABCs; and give cyanide antidote as ordered.

Notes: _____

Nerve Agents

Nerve agents are chemical agents that block nerve impulses causing paralysis. Example: Sarin gas in 1995 Tokyo subway attack.

- *Causes:* These agents can be absorbed through the skin or inhaled and block neuromuscular junction enzymes.
- *Signs and symptoms:* Remember SLUDGE (**S**aliva, **L**acrimation, **U**rination, **D**efecation, **G**I upset, and **E**mesis). Early symptoms include tachycardia; lethargy; paralysis; shock; anxiety; broncho-spasms; ataxia; and pulmonary edema.
- *Interventions:* Decontaminate the patient. If the agent was ingested orally, anticipate orders to give 1 g/kg of charcoal. Other orders may include atropine to reverse central nervous system effects; Atrovent (ipratropium) nebulizer to dry secretions; pralidoxime slowly over 30 minutes or obidoxime.

Notes: _____

Plague

Plague is a contagious bacterial infection (*Yersinia pestis*). Example: "Black Death" or "Great Plague" of the 14th century killed millions from Asia to Africa and Europe.

- *Causes:* This bacterial infection is found endemically in animals. It spreads directly by infected flea bites to humans and other animals. Its three types are bubonic, septicemic, and pneumonic.

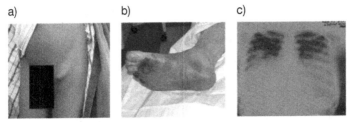

a) b) c)

Figure 5.2 Forms of plague: a) Bubonic plague, b) septicemic plague, c) pneumonic plague. *Source: www.cdc.gov/plague/symptoms/index.html*

- *Signs and symptoms (see Figure 5.2):*
    - Bubonic: Within 1 week, acute fever; chills; weakness; painful, swollen, lymph nodes (buboes).
    - Septicemic: Fever; chills; weakness; blackened necrotic extremities; abdominal pain; and sepsis.
    - Pneumonic: Fever; headache; weakness; dyspnea; hemoptysis; chest pain; rapid and severe pneumonia; respiratory failure; and shock. It is the only type that can be spread via droplets.
- *Interventions:* Droplet precautions; anticipate orders to obtain intravenous access; arrange for chest x-ray; arrange lymph node aspiration; collect blood and sputum cultures; and give antibiotics (streptomycin or gentamicin).

Notes: _____

Question: How is the plague most commonly transmitted to humans?
Answer: *By direct contact with infected rodent fleas.*

Q-Fever

Q-fever is a *Coxiella burnetii* bacterial infection. Complications may include hepatitis, myocarditis, and pneumonia.

- *Causes: Coxiella burnetii* bacteria found in animals and animal products (unpasteurized milk).
- *Signs and symptoms:* Within 2 to 3 weeks, the patient experiences flu-like symptoms (high fevers; cough; fatigue; nausea, vomiting, and diarrhea); abdominal pain; and chest pain.

- *Interventions:* Maintain standard precautions; anticipate orders to obtain complete blood count, liver enzymes, metabolic panel, chest x-ray, and cultures; and give antibiotics (doxycycline and ciprofloxacin).

Notes: _____

Radiation

Radiation is a natural or manufactured form of energy that can be dangerous at high levels of exposure.

- *Causes:* High-level exposures from sources such as a terrorist attack or nuclear power plant accident.
- *Signs and symptoms:* Burns; nausea, vomiting, and diarrhea; weakness; bleeding; confusion; sepsis; or symptom free.
- *Interventions:* Provide medical personnel with radiation detection devices; use reverse isolation/neutropenic precautions; anticipate orders to obtain a complete blood count, provide trauma/burn care, administer fluids intravenously, and give nausea medications and iodide tablets.

Notes: _____

Question: An ED patient significantly exposed to radiation on the job will have which symptoms?
Answer: *Bloody diarrhea, nausea, and vomiting within 3 hours of radiation exposure.*

Smallpox

Smallpox is a viral infection (*Variola major*).

- *Causes:* Spread by prolonged face-to-face contact; direct contact; or an exchange of bodily fluids.
- *Signs and symptoms:* Two to 3 days of fever; fatigue; nausea and vomiting; and delirium. This is followed by an approximately 4- to 6-mm macular rash on the face and extremities that turn to papules, vesicles, pustules, and finally scars (see Figure 5.3).

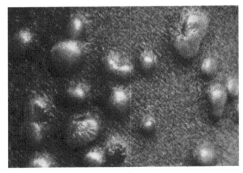

Figure 5.3 Smallpox rash. *Source: www.cdc.gov/smallpox/symptoms/index.html*

■ *Interventions:* Take airborne and contact precautions; place patient in negative pressure room; contact the CDC for laboratory testing and wound care; and give smallpox vaccination as ordered.

Notes: _____

Fast Facts in a Nutshell

Smallpox has been successfully eradicated as a result of multinational vaccinations. Because people are no longer vaccinated, there is concern that the *V. major* virus could be used as a bioterrorism weapon.

Tularemia

Tularemia is a gram-negative bacterial infection (*Franciscella tularensis*).

■ *Causes:* Spread by contact with infected animals, biting flies, or ticks.
■ *Signs and symptoms:* Within 2 weeks, the patient may experience abdominal pain; fever; nausea, vomiting, and diarrhea; pneumonia; conjunctivitis; skin ulcer; and lymphadenitis.
■ *Interventions:* Maintain standard precautions; gather blood, wound, or sputum cultures; and give antibiotics (ciprofloxacin, doxycycline, and gentamicin) as ordered.

Notes: _____

Viral Hemorrhagic Fevers

Viral hemorrhagic fevers include infections, such as Ebola, Marburg, and yellow fever.

- *Causes:* Spread by inhalation, direct contact, or bodily fluid exchange.
- *Signs and symptoms:* Within 3 weeks, the patient experiences fever; headache; weakness; diarrhea; vomiting; petechial rash; jaundice; bruising; hemorrhaging; disseminated intravascular coagulation; hepatitis; and renal failure.
- *Interventions:* Document travel history in past 21 days; establish airborne/contact precautions; place patient in negative pressure room; notify the hospital infection preventionist and the CDC; anticipate orders to obtain a complete blood count, liver function tests, prothrombin/partial thromboplastin time, and enzyme-linked immunosorbent assay (ELISA) testing; provide supportive treatment; and give antivirals, such as arenavirus or ribavirin. Scene safety always comes first. Medical personnel require full-body PPE and personal air-purifying respirators. *Take your time* to ensure proper donning and doffing techniques for highly infectious diseases using a buddy system and equipment checklist. Visit the CDC website to view recommended web-based PPE training. Only yellow fever vaccine is currently available, but the infection typically takes over before the vaccine is effective.

Notes: _____

Cholera (*Vibrio cholerae*)

Cholera, an intestinal infection caused by the bacterium *V. cholerae*, is uncommon in the United States, but may occur in individuals who return home after travel to Africa, India, or South America. Its severe effects can be life-threatening, from rapid loss of body fluids and shock. It is estimated that 100,000 people die annually from cholera.

- *Causes:* Spreads through ingested fecal-contaminated water or food.
- *Signs and symptoms:* Severe watery diarrhea and vomiting; leg cramps; dehydration; and shock.
- *Interventions:* Maintain standard precautions; anticipate orders to perform a complete blood count and basic metabolic panel;

provide fluid bolus intravenously; and possibly give antibiotics and zinc supplements.

Notes: _____

SUMMARY

Disasters are rarely predictable and are always chaotic. So, it is critical that you be prepared and know the plan of action for your facility. Become familiar with all available disaster equipment. Although this chapter should give you a good working knowledge of common forms of disasters and what to do, participating in disaster drills is an essential piece of the puzzle. Be sure to routinely refresh your disaster nursing skills by actively participating in regional drills and exercises.

6

Endocrine Emergencies

The endocrine system is made up of several complex hormone-secreting glands. These include the pituitary, pineal gland, hypothalamus, parathyroid, thyroid, pancreas, adrenals, testes, and ovaries. When one thinks of the endocrine system, the word that might come to mind is "hormones." While the endocrine system is responsible for hormone production, it also affects metabolism, growth and development, emotions, tissue function, and homeostasis. Although there are many endocrine-related illnesses, this chapter includes only the most common and emergent. After reviewing this chapter, you will be able to differentiate the different types of endocrine emergencies and their causes, manifestations, and treatments.

During this part of your orientation, locate and become familiar with:

- Blood glucose monitoring devices
- Diabetic ketoacidosis (DKA) policy and procedures
- Dietary supplies in your emergency department (ED)
- Medications to know: Insulin, insulin drips, antipyretics, beta-blockers, iodides, and propylthiouracil (PTU), oral and intravenous (IV) potassium, sodium bicarbonate, IV calcium, IV dextrose, glucagon, sodium polystyrene sulfonate (Kayexalate), and albuterol

PANCREATIC-RELATED EMERGENCIES

The pancreas is located in the mid-upper abdomen and is responsible for production and secretion of insulin and digestive enzymes such as amylase and lipase.

Diabetic Ketoacidosis (DKA)

DKA is a state of metabolic acidosis that is the result of elevated blood sugar (> 250 mg/dL). When the blood sugar is this high, the body does not have sufficient insulin to break down sugar for energy. To compensate, the body breaks down fat, thereby releasing toxic ketone acids.

- *Causes:* Uncontrolled blood sugar in diabetes mellitus, pancreatitis, and alcohol or drug abuse.
- *Signs and symptoms:* Dry, flushed skin; serum glucose level greater than 250 mg/dL; nausea and vomiting; abdominal pain; increased thirst; tachycardia; hypotension; urinary frequency; weakness; Kussmaul breathing; ketones in urine; change in level of consciousness; and coma.
- *Interventions:*
  - *Fluid replacement:* Administer IV normal saline bolus. Use caution if patient has a history of congestive heart failure or renal failure. Once you replace fluids, be prepared for urinary frequency. Provide urinals or bedpans. Collect urinalysis and monitor intake and output.
  - *Correct acidosis:* Check arterial blood gases; obtain beta-hydroxybutyrate (BHB) levels; monitor pulse oximetry or wave form capnography; administer IV sodium bicarbonate if ordered.
  - *Balance electrolytes:* Monitor anion gap, metabolic panel, cardiac rhythm; give nothing by mouth (NPO); medicate for nausea and vomiting. Anticipate IV potassium orders for hypokalemia. *Insulin administration drives potassium back into the cells, further reducing serum potassium levels.*
  - *Treat hyperglycemia:* Obtain and monitor hourly blood glucose, acetone level, and urinalysis; give insulin (first, 5–10 units of regular IV push, and then 0.1 units per kilogram per hour by IV fusion on a pump). Once the patient's blood sugar is less than 200 to 250 mg/dL, change from IV to subcutaneous insulin per the provider's order. IV 5% dextrose 0.45% normal saline (D5½NS) at a rate of 150 to 200 mL per hour

may be ordered as serum sodium returns to normal and glucose levels reach 250 mg/dL or less. Prepare for possible intensive care unit admission.

Notes: _____

Question: A 29-year-old diabetic female arrives who has dried skin, is flushed, is hot, and has Kussmaul respirations. What is the underlying illness?

Answer: *DKA—check her blood sugar.*

Question: When is DKA considered resolved?

Answer: *When the serum pH is greater than 7.3, serum bicarbonate level is greater than or equal to 18 mEq/L, blood glucose is less than 200 mg/dL, and anion gap is less than or equal to 12; corrections should be gradual to avoid cerebral edema.*

Question: How often should you check blood sugars on a patient receiving an insulin IV drip?

Answer: *Every hour.*

Hyperosmolar Hyperglycemic Syndrome (HHS)

This is a severe state of dehydration as a result of a very high blood sugar count (>600 mg/dL, but usually in the 1,000s). It is commonly associated with type 2 diabetes, recent surgery, or illness.

- *Causes:* The high level of sugar results in very thick blood, as the body tries to void the sugar. The process of frequent voiding, however, results in excessive loss of body fluids.
- *Signs and symptoms:* Imagine a shriveled, dried-up raisin, as this is your patient with hyperosmolar hyperglycemic syndrome (HHS). Look for thirst; warm and dry skin; dry mucosa; urinary frequency; weakness; change in level of consciousness; seizures; tachycardia; hypotension; fever; and absence of ketones in urine.
- *Interventions:*
  - *Fluid replacement:* These patients may need up to 9 to 12 L of IV fluids. Anticipate orders to start with normal saline IV bolus. Increased bolus rate may be ordered if hypotension is present. Frequently document vital signs. Use caution if patient has a history of congestive heart failure or renal failure. Once you

replace fluids, be prepared for urinary frequency. Provide urinals or bedpans. Collect urinalysis and monitor intake and output.

■ *Balance electrolytes:* Monitor serum osmolality, metabolic panel, and cardiac rhythm; obtain electrocardiogram; keep NPO; medicate for nausea and vomiting. Anticipate IV potassium orders for hypokalemia. *Insulin administration drives potassium back into the cells, further reducing serum potassium levels.*

■ *Treat hyperglycemia:* Obtain and monitor blood glucose hourly, acetone level, and urinalysis; give insulin (5–10 units of regular IV push, and then 0.05 units per kilogram per hour by IV fusion on a pump until blood sugar is less than 300 mg/dL). Goal is to reduce serum glucose by 50 to 70 mg/dL per hour. Once the patient's blood sugar is less than 200 to 300 mg/dL, change from IV to subcutaneous insulin per the provider's order. IV 5% dextrose 0.45% normal saline (D5½NS) at a rate of 150 to 200 mL per hour may be ordered as serum sodium returns to normal and glucose levels reach 250 mg/dL or less. Prepare for possible intensive care unit admission.

Notes: _____

Fast Facts in a Nutshell

Note the symptom and blood sugar differences between HHS and DKA.

■ Hyperosmolar hyperglycemic syndrome means that blood sugar is very high (600–1,000s mg/dL). It is more common in type 2 diabetics. Patient is severely dehydrated, serum pH is normal, and there are *no* ketones in the urine.

■ DKA blood sugar is moderately high (250–600 mg/dL). It is more common in type 1 diabetics or new onset. The patient may be mildly dehydrated, arterial blood gas (ABGs) reveal acidosis, and ketones are present in the urine.

Hypoglycemia

Hypoglycemia is defined as a low blood sugar (<60–70 mg/dL) and most commonly affects type 1 diabetics.

- *Causes:* Taking too much insulin or diabetic medication; lack of food intake; pancreatic tumor; sepsis; stress; pregnancy; alcohol ingestion; adrenal insufficiency; liver disease; and certain medications such as beta-blockers, nonsteroidal anti-inflammatory drugs (NSAIDs), and thyroid hormones.
- *Signs and symptoms:* Anxiety; hunger; sweating; dry mouth; pallor; altered mental status; confusion; lethargy; headache; hypothermia; loss of consciousness; and death.
- *Interventions:* Obtain accurate history, complete neurological assessment, and assess for cause of hypoglycemia. Anticipate orders to obtain blood glucose, monitor cardiac rhythm and vital signs, provide warm blankets and warming measures if hypothermic, obtain IV access, obtain complete blood count and metabolic panel, and recheck the blood glucose in 1 hour of treatment and as needed.
    - *If conscious:* Anticipate orders to give simple carbohydrates orally in the form of orange juice, soda, or glucose gel to quickly raise the blood sugar. Then give the patient a sandwich meal or regular diet tray to provide complex carbohydrates that will sustain the blood sugar.
    - *If unconscious:* Anticipate orders to give IV dextrose or intramuscular glucagon if unable to obtain IV access. Once patient regains consciousness, give simple carbohydrates followed by complex carbohydrates. *Vomiting may occur after glucagon administration; consider aspiration precautions.*

Notes: _____

Pancreatitis

This is the result of an increase in pancreatic enzymes. Whether it is caused by overproduction or obstruction, the enzymes erode or eat away the pancreatic tissues. Pancreatitis can spread to the liver, diaphragm, lungs, and other nearby organs. It is basically the pancreas in self-destruct or autodigestion mode.

- *Causes:* Alcohol abuse; gallstones; infections; injury; autoimmune disorder; and drug toxicity. Contributing factors include smoking, stress, and crash dieting or binge eating.
- *Signs and symptoms:* Midepigastric abdominal pain radiating to the back; diminished bowel sounds; nausea and vomiting;

abdominal distention; fever; jaundice if gallstones; weight loss; tachycardia; hypotension; frothy and foul-smelling stools; dark urine; Grey Turner's sign (see Figure 6.1); Cullen's sign (see Figure 6.2); and altered blood sugar.

- *Interventions:* Anticipate orders to administer fluids intravenously; monitor serum amylase, serum lipase, and blood glucose level; use nasogastric tube for decompression; administer nothing by mouth; give medications (antacids, anticholinergics, histamine receptor agonists, insulin, and analgesics/narcotics); prevent and treat infections; prepare for ultrasound or CT; prepare for possible surgery; and instruct patient on diet (low-fat diet, no caffeine, and no alcohol).

Notes: _____

Question: What is the normal serum amylase level in adults younger than 60 years?
Answer: *25 to 125 U/L.*

The patient who is actively vomiting cannot drink water before seeing the ED provider *in case the patient ends up going to surgery.*

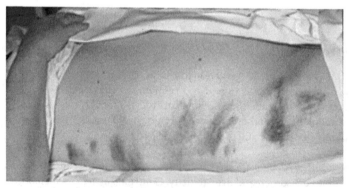

Figure 6.1 Grey Turner's sign. *Source: Photo by Herbert L. Fred and Hendrik A. van Dijk (Wikimedia Commons).*

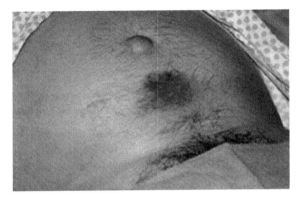

Figure 6.2 Cullen's sign. *Source: Photo by Herbert L. Fred and Hendrik A. van Dijk (Wikimedia Commons).*

THYROID-RELATED EMERGENCIES

The thyroid is located in the anterior aspect of the neck and affects calcium metabolism. Thyroid emergencies are rare, but can be life threatening.

Thyroid Storm

Thyroid storm is a life-threatening emergency that results from poorly managed hyperthyroidism.

- *Causes:* Uncontrolled hyperthyroidism. Risk factors include history of Graves' disease, medication noncompliance, trauma, infection, child birth, recent surgery, illness, or stress.
- *Signs and symptoms:* Vary, but may include: high fever; tachycardia; hypertension; vomiting; diarrhea; jaundice; thinning hair; weight loss; sweating; restlessness; exophthalmos; goiter; and tremors.
- *Interventions:* Obtain accurate history and list of medications; promptly manage any airway, breathing, and circulation concerns first; and provide supportive care. Anticipate orders to administer antipyretics, beta-blockers (propranolol), iodides, and PTU; obtain IV access; obtain serum thyroid function, metabolic panel, complete blood count, and toxicology screen; apply

cooling blankets for targeted temperature management; give supplemental oxygen; and obtain CT of head.

Notes: _____

Fast Facts in a Nutshell

A patient in thyroid storm may appear almost toxic with extremely high fevers reaching as high as 103° to 105°F. Treatment should be aggressive, as this a life-threatening emergency!

Myxedema Coma

Myxedema coma is a rare but emergent complication of uncontrolled or undiagnosed hypothyroidism. It is more common in women than in men and occurs more often in the winter months.

- *Causes:* Iodine deficiency; pituitary dysfunction; medications such as lithium, beta-blockers, amiodarone, narcotics, interferon, anticonvulsants, and general anesthesia; stress; burns; infection; surgery; trauma; and hypothermia.
- *Signs and symptoms:* Fatigue; shortness of breath; weight gain; generalized edema; constipation; pale cool skin; multiple organ dysfunction; hypothermia; bradycardia; bradypnea; confusion; depression; decreased urinary output; possible hypoglycemia; altered mental status or psychosis; coma; respiratory failure; and death.
- *Interventions:* Support airway, breathing, and circulation. Anticipate orders to obtain IV access; complete blood count, thyroid levels, metabolic panel, and serum creatinine levels; have electrocardiogram (EKG); administer IV or oral thyroxine (T4); slowly and passively rewarm patient; monitor intake and output; and administer analgesics and glucocorticoids.

Notes: _____

Fast Facts in a Nutshell

Be sure to closely monitor the cardiac rhythm of a myxedema coma patient. EKG findings associated with myxedema coma include bundle branch blocks, complete heart blocks, ST segment and T-wave changes, and bradycardia with prolonged QT intervals.

Question: Prolonged QT intervals can be a precursor for which type of arrhythmias?
Answer: *Ventricular tachycardia and torsades de pointes.*

SUMMARY

Those little hormones can affect so much more than just your mood. The endocrine system can affect multiple body systems. If you have ever been pregnant, you may have experienced just how much hormones can affect the rest of the body. Early recognition, thorough assessment, and rapid treatment are crucial to the survival of an endocrine-related emergency.

7

Environmental Emergencies

L et us face it, potential environmental hazards are all around us. The love of outdoor sports and activities contributes to the risks of environmental emergencies. Caring for the environmentally ill or injured patient is a common occurrence in the emergency department (ED). This chapter guides you through the many common types of environmental challenges you may face. Because no two environments are quite the same, be sure to become familiar with the most common environmental emergencies in your area.

During this part of your orientation, locate and become familiar with:

- Local and state animal bite-reporting regulations
- Wound cleansing or irrigation materials
- Tetanus vaccination policy and procedures
- Rabies vaccination policy and procedures
- Local and state assault-reporting procedures
- Venomous creatures indigenous to your area
- Poisonous plants indigenous to your area
- Hemostatic dressing material
- Operating room (OR) admission process
- Warming equipment
- Cooling equipment

BITES

Animal Bites

The most common animal bites seen in the ED are dog or cat bites. Occasionally, you may encounter a patient with a raccoon, rodent, or rabbit bite. Dog bites may cause more tissue damage, whereas cat bites pose a higher risk for infection.

- *Causes:* Break in the skin or tissue damage related to bite injury from an animal.
- *Signs and symptoms:* May range from lacerations, puncture wounds, to crush or soft tissue injuries.
- *Interventions:* Report all animal bites to your local animal control health authority. Assess wounds, noting any deformities or signs of infection. Anticipate orders to irrigate the wound with copious amounts of saline; administer antibiotics for high-risk injuries; administer rabies vaccine (only if the patient is unable to locate and quarantine the animal for 10 days); and administer tetanus vaccine if not vaccinated within past 5 years.

Notes: _____

Question: Which animal bite has the greatest risk for infection: dog, cat, or rat?
Answer: *Cat, because cats come in more contact with bacteria-infected rodents and create small puncture wounds.*

Question: A 36-year-old female comes in complaining of being bitten by a mouse. Should you give a rabies vaccine?
Answer: *No, small rodents do not carry rabies. However, skunks, foxes, raccoons, coyotes, dogs, cats, and bats may carry rabies.*

Question: If actually contracted, is rabies fatal without proper vaccination?
Answer: *Yes.*

Brown Recluse Spider

Brown recluse spiders are light brown with a darker brown violin-shaped mark on their backs (see Figure 7.1). Spider bites are actually

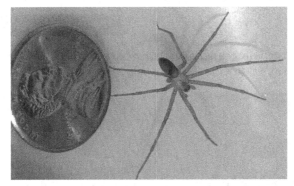

Figure 7.1 Brown reculse spider. *Source: Wikimedia Commons.*

pretty rare. Most spiders bite only when threatened. Nevertheless, many ED patients arrive almost daily, mistaking a common staph infection for a spider bite.

- *Causes:* Bite from a brown recluse spider.
- *Signs and symptoms:* Initial bite is usually painless. Brown recluse venom is cytotoxic and hemolytic. Basically, a bite from this spider may result in tissue necrosis. Most commonly, your patient will experience only some erythema and pain at the site. Rarely, the erythema then develops a red or bluish blood-filled blister. When this blister ruptures, it leaves a necrotic ulcer.
- *Interventions:* Anticipate orders to cleanse and dress the affected area and administer prophylactic antibiotics, analgesics, and tetanus vaccine. Most brown recluse bites heal without any medical attention. However, a small percentage of patients may develop a secondary infection.

Notes: _____

The bite of a brown recluse spider may cause skin ulcers (see Figure 7.2). An easy way to remember this is to spell ulcer backward!

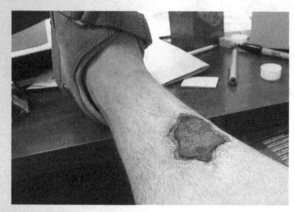

Figure 7.2 Skin ulcer. *Source: Photo by Jeffery Rowland (Wikimedia Commons).*

Black Widow Spider

Female black widow spiders are shiny black with a bright red hourglass mark on their abdomen (see Figure 7.3). Although the black widow's potent venom is neurotoxic, fatalities are rare. Children, elderly, and cardiac patients are more at risk.

- *Causes:* Bite from a black widow spider.
- *Signs and symptoms:* Muscle cramps; muscle contractions or spasms; musculoskeletal pain; severe abdominal pain similar to appendicitis; nausea; vomiting; hypertension; fever; weakness; headache; fatigue; anxiety; restlessness; and seizures. These symptoms may begin within a few hours and may last several days.
- *Interventions:* Treatment is usually supportive. Stabilize any airway, breathing, or circulation concerns first. Consult poison control and apply ice to the bite area to slow action of the venom. Anticipate orders to administer calcium gluconate, narcotics, muscle relaxants, and antivenom, if high-risk patient.

Notes: _____

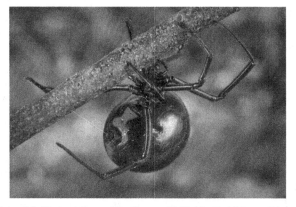

Figure 7.3 Black widow spider. *Source: CDC Public Health Image Library.*

Crocodile and Alligator Bites

Alligator and crocodiles are found in Africa, Asia, South America, Australia, and in the southern United States.

- *Causes:* Bites from alligators or crocodiles typically produce crushing, de-gloving injuries with multiple puncture wounds. In addition, a wide variety of bacteria can be found in the mouth of an alligator or crocodile. Therefore, these bites carry a high risk for infection.
- *Signs and symptoms:* Deep, severe soft tissue crush and de-gloving injury with multiple puncture wounds. Patient may also arrive with limb amputation and in a state of hemorrhagic or hypovolemic shock.
- *Interventions:* Assess and treat any uncontrolled external hemorrhage with direct pressure, hemolytic and/or compression dressings, and, if severe, tourniquets. Stabilize airway, breathing, and circulation issues. Anticipate orders to obtain two large-bore intravenous (IV) accesses, complete blood count (CBC) with differential, blood cultures, wound cultures, and type and crossmatch. Other orders may include administration of multiple broad spectrum IV antibiotics, intramuscular tetanus prophylaxis, IV crystalloid fluids, x-rays, splinting of deformed or fractured extremities, wound care/debridement, O-negative blood transfusion, and preparation for OR admission. Document repeated circulatory assessment findings before and after each intervention to determine effectiveness.

Human Bites

The human mouth carries more germs than that of most other animals. Therefore, a human bite is usually at a higher risk for infection than most animal bites.

- *Causes:* Bite from a human. You may see this if your patient was assaulted.
- *Signs and symptoms:* Bite marks to the skin resulting in puncture wounds, lacerations, soft tissue damage, crush injury, and, rarely, amputation.
- *Interventions:* Anticipate orders to irrigate, cleanse, and dress wound and administer prophylactic antibiotics such as Augmentin (amoxicillin clavulanate). Report assaults to your local police department according to your state law.

Notes: _____

Lizard Bites

- *Causes:* Bite from a lizard. Most lizard bites are nontoxic. However, Gila monsters (see Figure 7.4) and Mexican bearded lizards are venomous. These two lizards are commonly found in the southwestern United States and northwestern Mexico.
- *Signs and symptoms:* The bite may cause tissue trauma and crush injuries. The venom may produce pain, swelling, edema, nausea, vomiting, weakness, hemorrhage, tachycardia, hypotension, respiratory failure, syncope, shock, and possibly anaphylaxis.

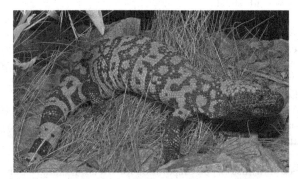

Figure 7.4 Gila monster. *Source: U.S. Fish & Wildlife Service, Arizona Ecological Services.*

- *Interventions:* Lizard antivenom currently does not exist. Stabilize any airway, breathing, or circulation problems first. Anticipate orders for wound care, administration of analgesics and tetanus prophylaxis, and supportive care.

Notes: _____

Shark Bites

- *Causes:* Bite from a shark. Most shark attack victims are taken by surprise and do not actually see what bit them. They often describe the attack as a sudden "tug" on an extremity. If you are working in an ED near the coastline, you need to be prepared to manage this injury.
- *Signs and symptoms:* Abrasions if the shark bumps the victim first; crescent-shaped bites; puncture wounds; shark teeth fragments; parallel scrapes or lacerations; bone fractures; tissue loss; amputations; hypothermia; and hypotension related to severe blood loss. (See also signs and symptoms of hypovolemic shock.)
- *Interventions:* Assess and control any external hemorrhaging first with direct pressure, hemostatic and/or pressure dressings, or a tourniquet, if severe. Stabilize airway, breathing, and circulation. Provide warmth, and apply oxygen. Anticipate orders to start two large-bore IV accesses, obtain blood type and crossmatch for possible blood transfusion, transfuse O-negative blood, and prepare for possible OR admission. Document repeated circulatory assessment findings before and after each intervention to determine effectiveness.

Notes: _____

Snakebites

Contrary to many movies, snakes are not usually aggressive creatures. They usually bite only if provoked or threatened. Snakes can be either venomous or nonvenomous. In the United States, there are only two types of venomous snakes: the pit vipers (rattlesnakes, copperheads, and cotton mouths) and the Elapidaes (coral snakes). Coral snake venom is neurotoxic, whereas pit viper venom is hemotoxic.

Fast Facts in a Nutshell

To quickly tell the difference between venomous and nonvenomous snakes, look at the shapes of their heads (see Figure 7.5). The rattlesnake on the left has a more triangular-shaped head than the nonvenomous garter snake on the right, which has a narrow round-shaped head.

Coral snakes are a little tricky (see Figure 7.6). You cannot really tell if they are venomous by the shape of the head. However, there is a rhyme some use to remember; it is based on the snake's bright red and yellow bands of color. "Red touching yellow kills a fellow." Or if "red touches black, venom lack."

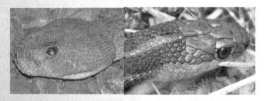

Figure 7.5 Rattlesnake (left) and garter snake (right). *Source: Wikimedia Commons (photo on right by Linda Tanner).*

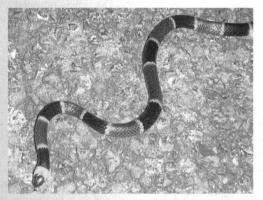

Figure 7.6 Coral snake. *Source: Wikimedia Commons.*

The first snakebite patient I cared for was a 6-year-old girl who was bitten by a baby copperhead. I saw firsthand how a snake could "play dead." When the adult accompanying the child poured the "dead" snake out of a coffee cup onto the counter, it began to wiggle all over the place. We could tell it was a baby copperhead right away by its bright green tail. The greatest concern with baby snakes is that they have not yet learned how to control the release of their venom. They are more likely to deliver all their venom in one bite, whereas the adult can control how much, if any, venom should be released. In this case, the child received a full dose of venom to her ankle. Due to her progressive systemic symptoms, she had to receive antivenom.

- *Causes:* Bite from a venomous snake.
- *Signs and symptoms:* Life-threatening reactions may include hypovolemic shock, respiratory failure, renal failure, and severe hemorrhage. Depending on the type of snake, your patient may experience the following:
  - *Local:* Bleeding; one or two puncture marks; redness; swelling; edema; tissue damage; possible tissue necrosis; and pain at the site.
  - *Systemic:* Nausea; vomiting; diarrhea; increased thirst; dizziness; diaphoresis; fever; syncope; paralysis; excessive salivation; speech difficulties; metallic or rubber taste; muscle twitching, paresthesia; gastric or rectal bleeding; epistaxis; hemoptysis; tachycardia; constricted pupils; oral swelling; abdominal pain; seizure; ecchymosis; petechiae; and weak pulse.
- *Interventions:* Stabilize airway, breathing, and circulation concerns first. Obtain an accurate history, including description of the snake, any treatment prior to arrival, time of bite, location, and number of bites. If the patient was bitten on his or her leg or arm, then immobilize affected limb at or below heart level and minimize exertion to reduce blood flow. Use a pen to mark a border of advancing edema every 15 minutes. Remove any jewelry or clothing from the bitten area. Anticipate orders to monitor cardiac rhythm, check blood pressure frequently, obtain large-bore IV access, administer IV crystalloid fluid bolus, administer analgesics for pain, administer tetanus prophylaxis, x-ray the affected area to reveal imbedded teeth, and obtain labs (complete blood count, electrolytes, blood urea nitrogen, creatinine, creatine phosphokinase levels, and type and crossmatch). Due to the cost and risk of anaphylactic reaction, antivenom is not usually given prophylactically. If your patient develops

worsening symptoms, coagulopathies, or major systemic reactions, such as hypotension or altered mental status, you may anticipate orders to administer antivenom such as CroFab.

Fast Facts in a Nutshell

Snakebite Management Myths—Corrected

Do *not* place a tourniquet above the site. When a tourniquet is taken off, it may release a venom bolus into the circulation, leading to systemic reaction.

Do *not* cut an "X" over the bite area and suck the venom out. It has been proven ineffective and may result in secondary infection.

Do *not* drink alcohol. Although drinking alcohol may lessen the patient's pain, it also dilates blood vessels, which may circulate the venom throughout the body faster.

Do *not* ice the limb. Although it may slow the blood flow to the area, icing is commonly associated with loss of a limb after a snakebite.

Believe it or not, most of your snakebite victims will try to kill the snake and bring it to show you which type of snake bit them. Educate your patients that a description of the snake will be safer for everyone.

Notes: _____

COLD-RELATED INJURIES

Frostbite

- *Causes:* Exposure to extreme cold.
- *Signs and symptoms:* Vary depending on temperature and length of exposure. Extent of tissue damage may not be evident until several days after exposure. Typically, the ears, nose, fingers, cheeks, and toes are affected first.
  - *First degree or "frostnip":* Involves superficial skin surfaces, itching, pain, tingling, pallor, or red patches. There is no permanent tissue damage.

- *Second degree:* Involves the skin and subcutaneous tissues, numbness, tingling, burning sensation, and stiff frozen skin. Upon thawing, frozen tissue may develop blisters, become mottled in color, and develop a hot stinging sensation.
- *Third degree:* Involves muscles, tendons, ligaments, and bones. Tissue may be white or pale yellow and waxy in appearance; tissues are cold and hard with lack of sensation to affected areas. As tissue thaws, blisters, edema of the extremity, and black-gray mottling may occur before gangrenous necrosis develops.
- *Interventions:* Rewarm the patient, monitor core temperature, and immerse affected areas in warm (104–110°F) water. Anticipate orders to administer pain medication, warm IV fluids; administer tetanus vaccine if needed; apply a warming blanket or just warm blankets; avoid friction or pressure to affected areas; dress thawed tissues with soft bulky dressings for protection; and elevate the affected area to reduce swelling. Teach patient that damage initially looks worse before it looks better and the healing process may take several months, depending on the damage.

Notes: _____

Fast Facts in a Nutshell

Thawing of frozen tissue is very painful. Avoid rubbing or using friction to warm frostbitten tissue, as this will increase tissue damage.

Hypothermia

Hypothermia is defined as a core temperature less than 95°F.

- *Causes:* Prolonged exposure to cold environment, submersion in cold water, and certain medical conditions such as hypoglycemia.
- *Signs and symptoms:* Shivering; weakness; slurred speech; confusion; weak pulses; bradycardia; dysrhythmias such as atrial or ventricular fibrillation; and bradypnea.
- *Interventions:* Anticipate orders to remove any wet clothing and dry the patient, cover the patient with warm dry blankets, monitor glucose levels, monitor core temperatures, monitor pulse oximetry and cardiac rhythm, increase room temperature, apply

warming blanket or use warming equipment available, infuse warmed IV fluids, and apply warmed humidified oxygen. If severe hypothermia, anticipate orders to use more active measures, such as warm peritoneal lavage, esophageal rewarming tubes, warm bladder irrigations, warm gastrointestinal irrigation, hemodialysis, continuous arteriovenous rewarming, and extracorporeal rewarming cardiopulmonary bypass.

Notes: _____

Question: What is the appropriate method for warming a shivering patient with a core temperature of 95°F (mild hypothermia)?
Answer: *Passive warming measures, such as warm environment, removal of wet clothes, and warm blankets.*

While you are trying to rewarm the hypothermic patient, something called "rewarming shock" may occur. As the patient begins to warm, peripheral vasodilation may occur, causing hypotension. As the cold blood from the extremities returns to the heart, it may further drop the core temperature and irritate the ventricles. This may lead to atrial or ventricular fibrillation.

Hypothermia may also cause oxygen to dissociate from hemoglobin, further reducing oxyhemoglobin concentrations.

NEAR DROWNING OR SUBMERSION EVENT

Near drowning is defined as surviving suffocation while submerged in a liquid. The term "drowning" results in death within 24 hours of a submersion event.

- *Causes:* Can be intentional or accidental. Drowning can also be secondary to a head/neck injury or cardiac event while in cold water. It is commonly seen in young children and toddlers.
- *Signs and symptoms:* May vary based on type of water or liquid, water temperature, length of submersion, concurrent injuries, and initiation of basic life support. Commonly you may see difficulty in breathing, tachypnea, or apnea, cold pale-blue or gray color skin, hypoxia, bradycardia, hypotension, dilated pupils or "fish eyes," vomiting, and hypothermia.

- *Interventions:* Treat any airway, breathing, or circulation concerns first, maintaining C-spine immobilization, as C-spine injuries are common with drowning victims. Anticipate orders to apply oxygen via nonrebreather or bag valve mask; prepare for intubation if necessary; monitor core temperature; monitor cardiac rhythm; perform EKG; establish IV access; remove wet clothing and warm the patient; obtain labs such as complete blood count, metabolic panel, and arterial blood gas.

Notes: _____

HEAT-RELATED INJURIES

Heat Exhaustion

- *Causes:* Prolonged exposure to warm temperatures and/or fluid loss without proper fluid and electrolyte replacement. If untreated, it may progress to heat stroke.
- *Signs and symptoms:* Extreme thirst; headache; dizziness; weakness; muscle cramps; nausea; vomiting; hypotension; tachycardia; fever; and syncope.
- *Interventions:* Place the patient on a stretcher and provide a cool, quiet area for the patient to rest. Anticipate orders to place the patient on a cardiac monitor, administer IV fluid bolus, monitor blood pressure and temperature, and possible application of cooling blanket. Discharge teaching should include measures to avoid or prevent future heat exhaustion.

Notes: _____

Heat Stroke

Heat stroke is a failure of the body to effectively dissipate heat and cool down. It is characterized by core temperatures over 105°F and can be fatal despite aggressive treatment.

- *Causes:* Prolonged exposure to hot temperatures, usually in combination with dehydration or physical exertion. Heat stroke can occur if children are locked in vehicles on hot days. Infants and the elderly are at increased risk. Risk factors include ingesting certain prescription or recreational drugs, preexisting medical conditions, high environmental temperatures, and high humidity.

- *Signs and symptoms:* Headache, dizziness, anxiety, and altered mental status; delirium; loss of muscle coordination; dilated/fixed pupils; seizures; hot, flushed, reddened, and dry skin; tachypnea; and coma.
- *Interventions:* Establish stable airway, breathing, and circulation first. Anticipate orders to apply oxygen, place patient on cardiac monitor, establish IV access, administer normal saline IV fluid bolus, cool the patient until core body temperature reaches 102°F, monitor core temperature frequently, administer corticosteroids if cerebral edema occurs, monitor intake and output, and prepare for possible intensive care unit admission. Cooling by evaporation with moistened skin may be more effective than with dry skin and application of cooling blanket. Applying padded ice packs to vascular areas (groin, axilla, and neck) also helps to quickly reduce core temperatures. Your goal is to avoid shivering, as it will increase your patient's oxygen consumption. If shivering occurs, anticipate orders to give 10 to 15 mg of chlorpromazine (Thorazine) intravenously.

Notes: _____

ROAD BURN OR ROAD RASH

Road burn/rash is a type of friction *abrasion*.

- *Causes:* Skin friction contact with the "road" or pavement or other abrasive material. It commonly occurs in motorcycle collisions, when the patient is not wearing protective gear.
- *Signs and symptoms:* Painful abrasions or large areas of skin that are "rubbed off." Imbedded debris or asphalt may be visible.
- *Interventions:* Treat any life-threatening injury first. Road rash is very painful; anticipate orders to apply local or topical anesthetics, or administer pain medication prior to wound cleansing with vigorous scrubbing. Once the local or topical anesthesia has had the desired effect, you will need to cleanse the wound, removing any debris. Personally, I like to use those surgical chlorhexidine scrub sponges with a sponge on one side and a soft brush on the other and normal saline to cleanse the wound. Next, you may

anticipate an order to apply antibiotic ointment and a nonadhesive dressing to the wounds.

Notes: _____

STABBINGS

- *Causes:* Forced penetration by a sharp object, commonly a knife.
- *Signs and symptoms:* Vary depending on the location, bleeding, tissue damage, organ damage, and signs of hypovolemic shock.
- *Interventions:* Note the size, length, and type of weapon used and location of injury; control bleeding with pressure and/or hemostatic dressing; monitor cardiac rhythm and blood pressure. Contact local law enforcement according to state law and hospital policy. Anticipate orders to start two large-bore IVs; obtain type and crossmatch for blood transfusion; give emergency blood transfusion, as ordered, if patient is in hypovolemic shock; and anticipate possible OR admission.

Notes: _____

STINGS

Hymenopteran stings (bees, fire ants, hornets, and wasps)

- *Causes:* Sting from hymenopteran venomous insects such as bees, fire ants, hornets, and wasps.
- *Signs and symptoms:* May vary from local reactions to severe systemic reactions depending on the location, number of stings, and patient sensitivity.
  - *Local:* Swelling, itching, redness, stinging, and burning.
  - *Systemic:* Edema, hives, bronchospasms, wheezing, and facial or oral swelling.
- *Interventions:* Treat any airway, breathing, or circulation problems first. Gently scrape stinger away with dull object (credit card), taking care not to squeeze the stinger, as it still contains some venom. Apply ice to site. Anticipate orders to administer antihistamines such as diphenhydramine (Benadryl) or famotidine (Pepcid), steroids such as methylprednisolone (Solumedrol), and, if severe, epinephrine 1:1,000 subcutaneously or

intramuscularly. Many patients who develop allergic reactions to bee stings receive a prescription for an EpiPen. Discharge teaching on proper use of the EpiPen is vital to reduce future risks of mortality from anaphylaxis.

Notes: _____

Question: When a patient arrives at the ED for a bee sting, which symptoms would alert the nurse that the patient needs emergent management?
Answer: *Angioedema, wheezing, or bronchospasms.*

Jellyfish Stings

- *Causes:* Sting from jellyfish. Be careful, because jellyfish that have washed ashore can still release venom.
- *Signs and symptoms:* Can be local or systemic and may vary based on size and type of jellyfish, duration of exposure, area of skin affected, age and health of the patient, and patient sensitivity.
  - *Local:* Instant stinging or burning; itching; tentacle print or patterned marks to the skin; numbness or tingling; and throbbing-type pain that may radiate up extremity. Jellyfish stings to the eye will require immediate eye irrigation and ophthalmology consult or follow-up.
  - *Systemic:* Headache; dizziness; fever; nausea; vomiting; muscle weakness; muscle spasm; joint pain; difficulty in breathing; arrhythmia; syncope; anaphylaxis; and cardiopulmonary arrest.
- *Interventions:* Treat any airway, breathing, or circulation problems first. Local reactions may be treated with topical antihistamines or corticosteroids. Anticipate orders to administer analgesics or topical anesthetics for pain, antihistamines, steroids, epinephrine, or, if box jellyfish, antivenom may be ordered.

Home remedies include rinsing the area with vinegar for at least 30 seconds to deactivate the venom. A paste made of seawater and baking soda has been known to deactivate venom of sea nettles and Portuguese man of war jellyfish. It is best to remove any tentacles with sea water, as freshwater may activate venom.

Notes: _____

Scorpion Stings

Scorpions are found primarily in the southwestern region of the United States. There are many different types, but only one whose neurotoxic venom is considered lethal. This deadly scorpion is none other than the *Centruroides sculpturatus*, more commonly known as the "bark scorpion," as it dwells on tree bark (see Figure 7.7).

- *Causes:* Sting from the tail of a venomous scorpion.
- *Signs and symptoms:* Commonly local and rarely systemic.
  - *Local:* Instant pain; edema; swelling; redness; and numbness or tingling. These symptoms usually resolve without treatment in a few hours.
  - *Systemic:* Agitation; anxiety; impaired speech; visual disturbances; incontinence; tachypnea; wheezing; stridor; excessive salivation; jaw muscle spasms; nausea; vomiting; hypertension; tachycardia; seizures; and anaphylaxis. These symptoms may last several days.
- *Interventions:* Support any airway, breathing, or circulation concerns first. Anticipate orders to treat the symptoms. These may include orders for ice pack to affected area, administration of analgesics or local anesthetics for pain, immobilization of the affected extremity to slow venom absorption, IV fluid bolus, antiemetics for vomiting, and/or antihistamines for swelling. The patient may need to be monitored for several hours to ensure there is no progression to a more severe reaction.

Notes: _____

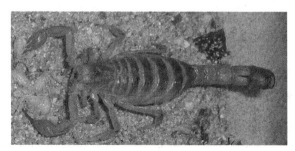

Figure 7.7 Scorpion. *Source: Wikimedia Commons.*

Stingray Stings

Stingrays are not typically aggressive creatures. They usually swim away if threatened. Most stings to humans are the result of a swimmer accidentally stepping on the back of the stingray.

- *Causes:* Sting from a stingray. If stepped on, the stingray instinctively whips its spikey venomous tail and may puncture the flesh of your patient (commonly on the leg). These spikes or spines may break off in the wound and continue to release venom.
- *Signs and symptoms:* May be local and/or systemic.
  - *Local:* Bleeding puncture wounds; lacerations; embedded spines; severe pain; muscle cramps; and swelling.
  - *Systemic:* Nausea; vomiting; diarrhea; headache; fever; chills; and hypotension.
- *Interventions:* Anticipate orders to place the affected area in warm water (about 113°F), taking care not to burn the patient. The warm water deactivates the venom and provides pain relief for the patient. The provider may also order local anesthetics, analgesics for pain, wound irrigation or debridement, prophylactic administration of antibiotics to prevent infection, and x-ray or ultrasound of the affected area to reveal any embedded barbs. The patient may require surgical exploration to remove all embedded barb fragments or spines. Prepare for possible OR admission. Preventive teaching should include teaching swimmers and divers to slide their feet across the ocean floor rather than stepping.

Notes: _____

Question: How long should the patient stung by a stingray soak his or her foot in hot water?
Answer: *Until the pain is relieved.*

SUMMARY

Environmental emergencies encompass a broad spectrum of injuries and illnesses. You may see one specific type of environmental emergency more than another, depending on your geographical area.

Taking the time to learn about the most common environmental emergencies unique to your location is vital. If you are new to the area, ask your colleagues or preceptor what to expect. Be sure to note the duration and location of exposure for any type of environmental illnesses or injuries. No matter which environmental emergency arises, be sure to educate your patients on prevention and protection against future environmental dangers.

8

Fluid and Electrolyte Imbalances

As you already may know, **fluid and electrolyte balance is essential to maintaining homeostasis within the body.** If not treated, interruptions to this balance can be fatal. Therefore, it is vital for the emergency department (ED) nurse to recognize the most common manifestations of fluid and electrolyte imbalances and how to correct them quickly.

During this part of your orientation, locate and become familiar with:

- Doppler machine for pedal pulses
- Peritoneocentesis tray and fluid containers
- IV fluids: Normal saline (0.9%) or 3% if severe, Ringer's lactate, dextrose 5% in water (D5W), and dextrose 5% in 0.45% normal saline (D5NS)
- Lab values: Sodium, potassium, calcium, phosphorus, magnesium
- Medications to know: Furosemide, potassium intravenously and by mouth, calcium chloride, calcium gluconate, sodium bicarbonate, magnesium sulfate, dextrose with intravenous (IV) regular insulin, sodium polystyrene sulfonate (Kayexalate), glucocorticoids, phosphate, calcitonin, and ethylenediaminetetraacetic acid

DIAGNOSES

Edema

Edema occurs when plasma fluid shifts into the interstitial space. There are four different types of edema based on location and injury.
Pulmonary edema: Fluid shifts to the lungs.

- *Causes:* Left-sided congestive heart failure; chest trauma; anaphylactic shock; and septic shock.
- *Signs and symptoms:* Shortness of breath; jugular vein distention (JVD); and crackle breath sounds.
- *Interventions:* Anticipate orders to arrange for chest x-ray, provide oxygen, and give diuretics (furosemide).

Notes: _____

Ascites: Fluid shifts to the abdomen.

- *Causes:* Liver problems or abdominal trauma.
- *Signs and symptoms:* Abdominal swelling/edema. The patient may also have pedal edema.
- *Interventions:* Anticipate patient will receive a peritoneocentesis and other measures to correct underlying liver problems.

Notes: _____

Pedal edema: Fluid shifts to the lower extremities.

- *Causes:* Right-sided congestive heart failure; lower extremity trauma; peripheral vascular disease; cast applied too tightly; high-sodium diet; and lymphedema.
- *Signs and symptoms:* Feet swelling and edema.
- *Interventions:* Give diuretic as ordered (furosemide); assess pedal pulses; and document stage of edema.

Notes: _____

Severe burns: Fluid shifts to burned areas, causing localized edema.

- *Causes:* The body's natural response to a severe burn injury: swelling and fluid shift.

- *Signs and symptoms:* Localized edema to burn area.
- *Interventions:* Volume replacement. Patient is experiencing cellular dehydration.

Notes: _____

Hyponatremia

Hyponatremia means that sodium level in the blood is less than 135.

- *Causes:* Syndrome of inappropriate antidiuretic hormone, medications (morphine sulfate, penicillin G, barbiturates, diuretics, and oxytocin), and too much D5W; nausea, vomiting, and diarrhea; gastrointestinal suction; excessive sweating; Addison's disease; extracellular fluid loss (burns, peritonitis, and bowel obstruction); and congestive heart failure.
- *Signs and symptoms:* Irritability; nausea and vomiting; seizures; weakness; hypotension; headache; tachycardia; lethargy; abdominal cramps; and dry oral mucosa.
- *Interventions:* Anticipate orders to correct fluid imbalances, intravenously administer normal saline 0.9% or 3% slowly if hyponatremia is severe, perform basic metabolic panel, and monitor closely. Goal is to change sodium levels at a rate less than or equal to 0.5 mEq/hr. Cerebral edema may occur if corrected too quickly.

Notes: _____

Hypernatremia

Hypernatremia is a condition with sodium level greater than 145.

- *Causes:* Diabetes insipidus; poor fluid intake in hot weather; fever; infections; renal disease; diarrhea; excessive sweating; diaphoresis; overly effective diuretics; and burns.
- *Signs and symptoms:* Anorexia; nausea; vomiting; agitation; thirst; oliguria; seizure; lethargy; coma; and muscle weakness/twitching.
- *Interventions:* Anticipate orders to give water by mouth or to start an IV line for IV rehydration.

Notes: _____

Hypokalemia

Hypokalemia is a condition with potassium level less than 3.5.

- *Causes:* Burns; gastrointestinal obstruction; acute alcoholism; diuretics; Cushing's syndrome (adrenal hyperactivity); nausea, vomiting, and diarrhea; uncontrolled diabetes mellitus; excessive sweating; or gastrointestinal suctioning.
- *Signs and symptoms:* Lethargy; fatigue; muscle weakness and decreased/absent deep tendon reflexes; tachycardia; paralysis; paralytic ileus; weak irregular pulse; tetany; orthostatic hypotension; and flatten/inverted T wave on an electrocardiogram.
- *Interventions:* Anticipate orders to correct alkalosis (no sodium bicarbonate, no vomiting, no diarrhea, and no gastrointestinal suctioning), administer potassium by mouth or intravenously, perform basic metabolic panel, check magnesium, and give IV lactated Ringer's fluids.

Notes: _____

Fast Facts in a Nutshell

- The correct infusion rate of an IV potassium drip is no faster than 20 mEq of potassium chloride per hour on a pump. Preferred dose is 10 mEq/hr.
- If infused too quickly, potassium drip can cause fatal arrhythmias and phlebitis!

Hyperkalemia

Hyperkalemia is a condition in which potassium level is greater than 4.5.

- *Causes:* Renal failure; diabetes mellitus; crush injury; early burn stages; aldosterone deficiency; excessive potassium intake; potassium-sparing diuretics; hyponatremia; and respiratory/metabolic acidosis.
- *Signs and symptoms:* Muscle weakness, cramps, and pain; dyspnea; peaked T waves and depressed ST segments on electrocardiogram; nausea, vomiting, and diarrhea; paresthesia; irritability; dysrhythmias; sinus bradycardia; first-degree heart block; ventricular fibrillation; and asystole.

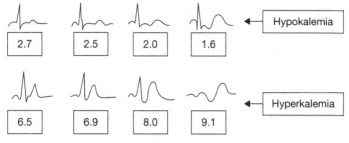

Figure 8.1 EKG changes in potassium imbalances.

- *Interventions:* Anticipate orders to monitor cardiac performance; restrict potassium intake (in food or medication); administer normal saline bolus intravenously; give diuretics, Kayexalate by mouth or rectum, and possibly albuterol nebulizer. When IV medications are ordered, give (IV) calcium chloride or calcium gluconate slow push over 5 minutes first to protect the heart, then IV glucose (dextrose 50% injection [D50]), then IV regular insulin, and finally IV sodium bicarbonate.

Figure 8.1 illustrates electrocardiogram changes during hypokalemia and hyperkalemia. You can see how potassium directly affects the heart.

Notes: _____

Fast Facts in a Nutshell

- It is normal to have a high potassium level with high blood sugar.
- As the blood sugar decreases with insulin treatment, the potassium will shift into the cell, and the serum potassium level will drop.

Hypocalcemia

Hypocalcemia is a condition in which calcium level is less than 8.5. It leads to increased neuromuscular excitability.

- *Causes:* Hypoparathyroidism; vitamin D deficiency; peritonitis; bone cancer; calcium channel blocker overdose; pancreatitis; burns; renal failure; sepsis; shock; citrate (anticoagulant used in blood transfusions); trauma; alcoholism; and malnutrition.

- *Signs and symptoms:* Anxiety; irritability; seizure; nausea, vomiting, and diarrhea; muscle cramps; tetany; dysrhythmias; unconsciousness; and cardiac failure.
  - Chvostek's sign: Facial muscle spasms when facial nerve tapped anterior to external ear below the temporal bone.
  - Trousseau's sign: Hand/carpal spasms when pumping up blood pressure cuff above systolic pressure for 3 minutes.
- *Interventions:* Anticipate orders to administer normal saline intravenously, monitor cardiac performance, give calcium chloride or calcium gluconate intravenously, and correct magnesium deficit.

Notes: _____

Hypercalcemia

Hypercalcemia is a condition with calcium level greater than 10.6. It leads to decreased neuromuscular excitability.

- *Causes:* Renal disease; hyperparathyroidism; too much vitamin D; drinking too much milk; pancreatitis; peptic ulcers; thiazide diuretics; and prolonged immobilization.
- *Signs and symptoms:* Muscle weakness; dehydration; nausea and vomiting; constipation; ileus; kidney stones; lethargy; headache; irritability; decreased level of consciousness; dysrhythmias (short QT interval); and cardiac arrest.
- *Interventions:* Anticipate orders to administer diuretics and 1 to 2 L of normal saline bolus intravenously, monitor cardiac rhythm, perform basic metabolic panel, measure magnesium level, measure intake and output, monitor for cardiac heart failure, and administer medications (glucocorticoids, calcitonin, phosphate, or ethylenediaminetetraacetic acid).

Notes: _____

Fast Facts in a Nutshell

To remember symptoms of hypercalcemia, just use the following rhyming words: moans, groans, bones, stones, and psych overtones.

Hypomagnesemia

Hypomagnesemia is a condition in which serum magnesium level is less than 1.7 mEq/L.

- *Causes:* May include malnutrition, alcoholism, cirrhosis, ulcerative colitis, diabetic ketoacidosis, diuretics, or renal disease.
- *Signs and symptoms:* Weakness; lethargy; hypotension; bradycardia or dysrhythmias (torsades de pointes); increased deep tendon reflexes; nausea; vomiting; coma; bradypnea; and may lead to cardiac or pulmonary arrest.
- *Interventions:* Anticipate orders to administer PO or IV magnesium, apply cardiac monitor, monitor vital signs, assess deep tendon reflexes, and monitor intake and output and magnesium levels. IV magnesium has multiple indications with various IV drip rates. Be sure to become familiar with the concentrations available to you; do not give IV magnesium too fast or your patient could go into cardiopulmonary arrest.

Notes: _____

Fast Facts in a Nutshell

IV magnesium has many doses that vary according to indication:

- For cardiac arrest due to hypomagnesemia or torsades de pointes, give 1 to 2 g diluted in 10 mL of D5W IV/intraosseous (IO).
- For torsades de pointes with a pulse or acute myocardial infarction with hypomagnesemia, give 1 to 2 g diluted in 50 to 100 mL D5W over 5 to 60 minutes IV.
- For hypomagnesemia, give 1 g diluted in 50 mL D5W over 30 to 60 minutes IV.

Hypermagnesemia

Hypermagnesemia is a condition in which serum magnesium level is greater than 2.3 mEq/L.

- *Causes:* May include magnesium overdose, renal disease, or adrenocortical insufficiency.

- *Signs and symptoms:* Lethargy; nausea; headache; diminished or absent deep tendon reflexes; muscle weakness or paralysis; bradypnea or apnea; hypotension; hypocalcemia; EKG changes; and cardiac or respiratory arrest.
- *Interventions:* Anticipate orders to monitor cardiac rhythms, deep tendon reflexes, vital signs, and magnesium levels; to administer calcium chloride or furosemide (Lasix) with saline diuresis. If severe, dialysis may be ordered.

Notes: _____

Overhydration

Overhydration is also known as "fluid overload."

- *Causes:* Drinking too much water or fluids. Receiving too much IV fluid and overproduction of antidiuretic hormone.
- *Signs and symptoms:* Pedal/pulmonary edema; nausea and vomiting; headache; anorexia; confusion; seizure; aphasia; or blurred vision.
- *Interventions:* Anticipate orders to restrict fluids, give diuretics, monitor and document intake and output, and document level of consciousness.

Notes: _____

Dehydration

Dehydration is a lack of fluids.

- *Causes:* Inadequate fluid intake; fever; diuresis; excessive sweating; burns; third spacing (internal bleeding, crush injury); and vomiting or diarrhea. Geriatrics and pediatrics are high-risk populations.
- *Signs and symptoms:* Confusion; disorientation; seizure; dry oral mucosa; dry skin; hyperthermia; weak rapid pulse; orthostatic hypotension; lethargy; fever; thirst; sunken fontanelles and eyes in infants; lack of tears in crying children; concentrated urine; tachypnea; tachycardia; and decreased urine output.
- *Interventions:* Anticipate orders to give fluids intravenously or by mouth, administer antipyretics for fever, perform basic metabolic

panel and EKG, document mental status, check orthostatic vital signs, and measure intake and output.

Notes: _____

SUMMARY

Fluids and electrolytes play a key role in health and homeostasis. It is critical that ED nurses understand this delicate balance, as a slight disturbance in this amazing balance can be fatal. Make sure you learn the different lab values, for you will need them every day in evaluating a wide variety of illnesses.

9

Gastrointestinal Emergencies

The gastrointestinal (GI) system is made up of several organs, including the stomach, liver, pancreas, gallbladder, and intestines. GI emergencies can be a very messy everyday emergency department (ED) occurrence. Ruptured bowels, vomiting, diarrhea, constipation, enemas, you name it; you will see all types of GI problems in the ED. Catching the projectile vomit in the basin is the real trick! After reviewing this chapter, you will be able to differentiate the types of GI emergencies, their causes, manifestations, and treatments. **For each patient, prepare a full GI assessment and document it thoroughly.**

During this part of your orientation, locate and become familiar with:

- Suction equipment
- Gastric lavage equipment and nasogastric tubes
- Hemoccult and gastroccult specimens
- Enemas
- Basins, Chux, and incontinence pads or liners
- Medications to know: GI cocktail, famotidine (Pepcid), pantoprazole (Protonix), promethazine (Phenergan), metoclopramide (Reglan), and ondansetron hydrochloride (Zofran)

NEVER UNDERESTIMATE ABDOMINAL PAIN

I once had a female patient come in by ambulance complaining of abdominal pain for 5 minutes. I thought it was a little silly to call an ambulance after just 5 minutes of pain. She was hollering, wailing, and carrying on so much that I could barely get a history. She was seen, assessed by a doctor, and x-rayed in about 15 minutes. Then she said her chest hurt. It turned out she not only had a ruptured bowel, but she also was having an acute myocardial infarction at the same time! Boy, we were shocked! So, although a patient may appear to be just very dramatic, **never underestimate abdominal pain.**

Fast Facts in a Nutshell

- A patient who has vomited 20 times in the past 8 hours is at risk for *metabolic alkalosis and hypokalemia* (see Chapter 8).
- After ingesting bleach, the patient has corrosive injury to the esophagus. Initial assessment and treatment should include *airway management*.
- Causes of ascites include *constrictive pericarditis, cirrhosis, and peritonitis.*
- *Sepsis* is the most common problem associated with colon trauma.

Question: The abdomen is assessed in which order?
Answer: *Inspection, auscultation, percussion, and palpation (look, listen, and feel).*

DIAGNOSES

Gastritis

Gastritis is an inflammation of the stomach lining that can be an acute or chronic condition. Chronic gastritis can lead to ulcers and GI bleeding.

- *Causes:* Infection; stress; acute illness; gastroesophageal reflux disease (GERD); aspirin; nonsteroidal anti-inflammatory drugs (NSAIDs); alcohol; or food poisoning.

- *Signs and symptoms:* Nausea and vomiting; gastric mucosal bleeding; epigastric pain; malaise; anorexia; and loss of appetite.
- *Interventions:* Anticipate orders to administer fluids intravenously, arrange for abdominal x-ray, provide blood if blood loss is severe, prepare a complete blood count; *H. pylori* testing; amylase level; lipase and basic metabolic panel; and administer medications (e.g., antacids, GI cocktail, histamine receptor antagonists, and antiemetics). Discharge teaching should include lifestyle modifications of six small meals daily, smoking cessation, and prescribed use of antacids.

Notes: _____

Fast Facts in a Nutshell

A GI cocktail is made up of a liquid antacid and belladonna alkaloids/phenobarbitol (Donnatal). (Adding 10 mL of viscous lidocaine makes it a super GI cocktail.)

Question: A 36-year-old male patient complains of burning epigastric pain 1 to 2 hours after eating, for 1 to 2 weeks. What is his diagnosis?
Answer: *Peptic ulcer disease.*

Gastroenteritis

Gastroenteritis is an inflammation of the stomach or small intestine. It is often the diagnosis when the patient says, "I think I have the stomach flu."

- *Causes:* Viruses; bacteria; parasites; toxins; or allergens. The most common viruses that cause gastroenteritis are Norwalk virus and rotavirus.
- *Signs and symptoms:* Nausea, vomiting, and diarrhea; abdominal pain or cramps; fever; dehydration; and hypovolemia in the very young or very old.
- *Interventions:* Practice strict handwashing and contact precautions; anticipate orders to provide fluids intravenously, prepare a basic metabolic panel and complete blood count, administer

medications (antibiotics and antiparasitic agents), and provide patient education on a clear liquid and BRAT (bananas, rice, applesauce, and toast) diet.

- Discharge teaching should include avoiding meat and dairy products, spicy foods, alcohol, greasy foods, and acidic foods.
- Infants should not stop formula feeding for more than 24 hours.
- Recovering from nausea and vomiting is a gradual process. The patient should have nothing by mouth for an hour or so after vomiting. Then clear liquids should be introduced in small increments (ice chips) for 24 hours, after which the patient can advance to full liquids. The next step is the BRAT diet; finally, the advanced diet as tolerated. Follow this process gradually or you will be cleaning up vomit!

Notes: _____

Gastroesophageal Reflux Disease (GERD)

GERD is commonly called "acid reflux." It occurs when excess stomach acid travels up the esophagus, resulting in esophagitis.

- *Causes:* The malfunction of the esophageal sphincter and hiatal hernia are the major causes. Contributing factors are cigarette smoking; lying down after meals; stress; pregnancy; medications; and consuming alcohol, large meals, spicy or acidic food, and caffeine. Complications such as scar tissue, dysphagia, and esophageal strictures may result from repeated exposure to gastric content.
- *Signs and symptoms:* Upper midsternal burning pain and indigestion that worsens with lying down.
- *Interventions:* Anticipate orders for barium swallow, antacids, and GI cocktail. Educate the patient to avoid fatty or fried foods, chocolate, alcohol, and overeating. The patient should drink plenty of water and avoid lying down for 3 hours after eating.

Notes: _____

Intestinal Obstruction

This is a potentially life-threatening condition resulting in the inability to move GI contents through the intestines. Your patient may present with severe pain and appear anxious. There are two types of obstructions: large bowel and small bowel. If you had to choose, you might prefer the large bowel obstruction, because nothing is coming out of either end. On the other hand, the patient with small bowel obstruction will be continually vomiting and having diarrhea. You will need plenty of bedpans and emesis basins.

- *Causes:* Previous abdominal surgery, adhesions; hernia; strictures; foreign bodies; volvulus (twisting of bowel); intussusception; tumor; paralytic ileus; mesenteric infarction; and abdominal angina.
- *Signs and symptoms:* Fever; abdominal distention; nausea and vomiting; rapid onset of severe abdominal pain; dehydration; weight loss or weight gain (due to fluid retention); high-pitched or absent bowel sounds; diaphoresis; weakness; restlessness; and constipation or recent diarrhea.
- *Interventions:* Anticipate orders to arrange for abdominal CT scan, ultrasound, or x-rays; monitor vital signs; give nothing by mouth; obtain complete blood count and metabolic panel; administer fluids intravenously, antiemetics and analgesics; insert nasogastric tube for gastric decompression; administer antibiotic medications; and prepare for possible operating room (OR) admission.

Fast Facts in a Nutshell

Tips for nasogastric tube insertion:

- Be nice when inserting a tube down a patient's *belly;* use lidocaine *jelly* to lubricate the tip.
- Apply oral anesthetic spray to the throat.
- Check placement initially by *auscultating stomach, confirming that the patient is able to speak, and checking gastric content.*
- To help the tube curve down the nasopharynx, curl the tip of the nasogastric tube around your finger first.

Notes: _____

Appendicitis

Appendicitis is an inflammation of the appendix. If it ruptures, it could lead to peritonitis, sepsis, and then septic shock!

- *Causes:* Unknown, but may be attributed to stomach virus, twisting, or obstruction of the appendix.

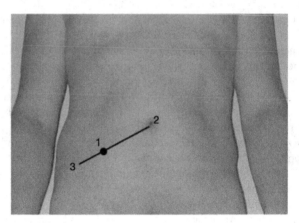

Figure 9.1 McBurney's point.

- *Signs and symptoms:* Constant dull right lower quadrant abdominal pain (McBurney's point; see Figure 9.1); rebound tenderness; nausea and vomiting; low-grade fever (usually after first 24 hours); and manifestations of peritonitis (fever, guarding, abdominal pain and distention, hypoactive bowel sounds, and diffuse rigidity).
- *Interventions:* Anticipate orders to give patient nothing by mouth (NPO), analgesics, antibiotics, antiemetics, and fluids intravenously. Arrange for a complete blood count, metabolic panel, type and screen, an abdominal CT scan or ultrasound, and possible surgery.
  - A patient sent to surgery should have a completed preoperative checklist and be wearing only a gown. There should be *no body jewelry in unusual places, no hearing aids, no dentures, no hairpins, no socks, no underwear—just a patient gown.*

Notes: _____

Esophageal Obstruction

Esophageal obstruction, or food bolus, is a term for food or foreign bodies that get stuck or lodged in the esophagus. Meats such as steak, pork, and poultry can easily become lodged in the esophagus. This may be why some refer to esophageal obstruction as the "steakhouse syndrome."

- *Causes:* Ingestion of a foreign object or simply not chewing well before swallowing. Other conditions pose an increased risk for esophageal obstruction, such as esophageal cancer, eosinophilic esophagitis, nutcracker esophagus, peptic strictures, and Schatzki rings.
- *Signs and symptoms:* Foreign body sensation: "I have something stuck in my throat." The patient may also have acute dysphagia, chest pain, neck pain, pain with swallowing, regurgitation of food, and drooling.
- *Interventions:* Treat any airway concerns first. Anticipate orders to obtain x-rays of the chest and soft tissue films of the neck, administer intravenous glucagon to relax esophageal smooth muscles, or prepare for endoscopy to retrieve the object. Patient discharge teaching should include chewing food thoroughly and use of dentures if applicable.

Notes: _____

Esophageal Varices (Bleeding)

Esophageal varices are enlarged or varicosed veins located in the lower part of the esophagus.

I will never forget the night I first cared for a patient with bleeding esophageal varices. He was a young man in his 40s, who came in via ambulance in full-fledged hypovolemic shock! His wife stated he was an alcoholic. He was as pale as the bed sheet beneath him, hypotensive, diaphoretic, tachycardic, semiconscious, and vomiting copious amounts of bright red blood. We had 3 units of O-negative blood rapidly infusing when the OR team arrived to perform an emergency endoscopic procedure right on the spot! The doctor finally was able to tie off the bleeding esophageal vessel. The patient was later admitted to the intensive care unit and developed disseminated intravascular coagulation due to massive blood loss. At the time, I had never imagined one could lose so much blood from a ruptured esophageal varice.

- *Causes:* Liver damage can lead to poor circulation through the portal vein, causing blood to back up into surrounding smaller vessels, such as esophageal veins. These fragile thin veins in the esophagus can then burst or rupture and bleed out into the esophagus. Other causes include thrombus, infection, and damage from liver cirrhosis.

- *Signs and symptoms:* Vomiting bright red blood, or dark and tarry stools. In severe cases, your patient may go into hemorrhagic/hypovolemic shock and require one-to-one monitoring.
- *Interventions:* Don necessary personal protective equipment (PPE) and treat any airway emergencies first. Anticipate orders to administer oxygen, beta-blockers such as propranolol, and medications to decrease portal vein pressure (octreotide, somatostatin, or vasopressin and nitroglycerin); insert large-bore intravenous access; monitor vital signs; assess and treat patient for any signs of hypovolemic shock; obtain type and crossmatch for possible blood transfusion; insert balloon tamponade; and prepare for endoscopy.

Notes: _____

Cholecystitis

Cholecystitis is an inflammation of the gallbladder.

- *Causes:* Gallstones; obstruction; or acute inflammation.
- *Signs and symptoms:* Right upper quadrant abdominal pain radiating to back or right shoulder that becomes worse after eating fatty foods; low-grade fever; clay-colored stool; nausea and vomiting; anorexia; flatulence; possible jaundice; fat intolerance; and Murphy's sign.
- *Interventions:* Anticipate orders to obtain gallbladder ultrasound, complete blood count, liver enzymes, HIDA scan, and abdominal CT; give nothing by mouth (NPO); administer fluids intravenously; give medications (analgesics, antibiotics, sedatives for smooth muscle relaxation, and antiemetics for nausea and vomiting); and use nasogastric tube for gastric decompression. Arrange for possible surgical intervention.
  - *Morphine sulfate should be avoided.* It can cause gallbladder spasms.
  - *Murphy's sign* is an increased sharp right upper quadrant abdominal pain that occurs during inspiration when palpating the patient's gallbladder and asking the patient to take a deep breath.
  - To palpate the gallbladder, press the fingers under the right anterior rib cage.

Notes: _____

GI Bleeding

GI bleeding can be classified as upper or lower. Patients with GI bleeding have a distinct odor. Once you have learned it, you can identify a patient with GI bleeding a mile away!

Upper GI Bleeding

- *Causes:* Esophageal varices; peptic ulcer; stomach cancer; alcohol abuse; and trauma.
- *Signs and symptoms:* Weakness, hypotension, hypovolemic shock, nausea and vomiting; bright red to coffee ground color emesis; and black tarry stools or dark-red rectal bleeding.
- *Interventions:* Anticipate orders to start an 18- or 16-gauge intravenous access; prepare a complete blood count—hemoglobin and hematocrit, metabolic panel, and coagulation studies; arrange for abdominal CT scan; insert nasogastric tube; document gastric content findings; assess guaiac gastric contents and stool; administer fluids intravenously; give histamine antagonists; test blood for type and crossmatch; and prepare for possible blood transfusion or endoscopy.

Lower GI Bleeding

- *Causes:* Internal or external hemorrhoids; constipation; polyps; diverticulitis; colon cancer; and irritable bowel syndrome.
- *Signs and symptoms:* Bright red rectal bleeding.
- *Interventions:* Anticipate orders to open large-bore intravenous access, prepare a complete blood count and coagulation studies, arrange for abdominal CT scan, assess guaiac gastric contents and stool, administer fluids intravenously, test blood for type and crossmatch, reverse coagulopathies, and prepare for possible blood transfusion.

Notes: _____

Fast Facts in a Nutshell

- Ulcerative colitis and Crohn's disease are inflammatory disorders of the colon and rectal mucosal lining. They can cause diffuse rectal bleeding.
- Ingesting bismuth subsalicylate (Pepto-Bismol), iron, and charcoal results in dark/black stools similar to those seen in upper GI bleeding.

Question: Your patient arrives with a history of alcohol abuse and cirrhosis. He is vomiting copious amounts of bright red blood. Vital signs are as follows: Blood pressure of 82/56, pulse of 144, respirations of 36, and temperature of 99.8°F. What do you do first?

Answer: *Suction blood from the airway (remember airway, breathing, and circulation [ABCs] first).*

SUMMARY

GI emergencies are daily events in the ED. You should now be able to differentiate the various types of GI emergencies. Be sure to assess, reassess, and document these patients carefully. Abdominal pain may involve a serious problem. Consider the cause of the patient's symptoms and manage pain in a timely manner.

10

Genitourinary Emergencies

Genitourinary emergencies are routinely seen and treated in the emergency department (ED). Most of the time they are minor problems that can be treated with medications. **However, genitourinary problems, such as testicular torsion, can result in loss of the testicle(s) if untreated.** This chapter guides you through the genital and urinary problems commonly faced in the ED. After reviewing this chapter, you will understand the causes, manifestations, and interventions for common genitourinary emergencies.

During this part of your orientation, locate and become familiar with:

- Different types of Foley and straight catheters
- Bladder irrigation systems
- Condom catheters
- Urine collection supplies
- Urinals
- Coudé catheter

DIAGNOSES

Urinary Tract Infection

This is a bacterial infection of the bladder and urethra.

- *Causes:* Because of their anatomy, urinary tract infections are more common in women than in men. Other contributing factors are holding your urine, not drinking enough water, intercourse, "kidney stones," and pH imbalances.

- *Signs and symptoms:* Painful urination (dysuria); hematuria; frequency; urgency; cloudy urine; foul-smelling urine; fever; and abdominal pain.
- *Interventions:* Obtain clean-catch urine or catheterized urine if vaginal bleeding is present, administer antibiotic as ordered, encourage fluids such as cranberry juice and water, discourage caffeinated drinks, discourage bubble baths, encourage sitz baths, teach to wipe from front to back after toileting, and teach sexually active females to void and cleanse perineal area after intercourse. If administering phenazopyridine, indicate that it will turn the urine orange and permanently stain underwear.

Notes: _____

PYELONEPHRITIS

This is a bacterial infection of the kidney or renal pelvis.

- *Causes:* Pyelonephritis usually starts as a urinary tract infection in the urethra or bladder that travels all the way up to the kidneys.
- *Signs and symptoms:* Flank pain; painful urination (dysuria); hematuria (macro or micro); frequency; urgency; cloudy urine; foul-smelling urine; fever; chills; costovertebral (CVA) tenderness, and nausea and vomiting. Urinalysis may reveal elevated white blood cell counts, nitrates, elevated red blood cell counts, and bacteria.
  - *Chronic pyelonephritis* (renal failure): Urine output less than 30 mL/hr (oliguria); elevated blood urea nitrogen and creatinine; hypertension; rapid weight gain; and altered loss of consciousness.
- *Interventions:* Obtain clean-catch urine or catheterized urine if vaginal bleeding is present, intravenous (IV) fluids, and antibiotic/antipyretics/antiemetics as ordered; encourage fluids such as cranberry juice and water, discourage caffeinated drinks, discourage bubble baths, encourage sitz baths and bed rest, teach females to wipe from front to back after toileting, and teach sexually active females to void and cleanse perineal area before and after intercourse.

Notes: _____

Renal Calculi

Renal calculi are stones of various sizes along the urinary tract that are commonly known as "kidney stones." The pain that they cause is equal to that experienced during childbirth!

- *Causes:* Kidney stones are usually made of calcium or uric acid salt deposits, possibly resulting from urine that is too alkaline or too acidic.
- *Signs and symptoms:* Severe flank pain radiating to the groin; nausea and vomiting (NV); hematuria; oliguria; pallor; diaphoresis; low-grade fever; and guarding.
- *Interventions:* Anticipate orders to: obtain clean-catch or catheter urine if vaginal bleeding is present; start IV line; administer analgesics (IV ketorolac) and document effectiveness; administer antiemetic medications; instruct to strain all urine; and prepare for CT scan of abdomen/pelvis without contrast. Do not forget to send patient home with a urine strainer.

Notes: _____

Epididymitis

Epididymitis is an intrascrotal infection.

- *Causes:* Sexually transmitted diseases or urinary tract infections.
- *Signs and symptoms:* Penile discharge, bacteria in urinalysis, gradual scrotum pain, fever, epididymis swelling, and chills.
- *Interventions:* Anticipate orders for ice pack to the scrotum, gonorrhea and chlamydia (G & C) culture, antibiotics; and instruct to abstain from sexual intercourse until follow-up repeat negative culture obtained.

Notes: _____

Fast Facts in a Nutshell

When preparing ceftriaxone (Rocephin) intramuscular (IM) injection, 1% lidocaine may be used as a diluent to decrease discomfort. Check for allergies to cephalosporins and lidocaine.

Testicular Torsion

This occurs when a testis spontaneously twists one or more times on the cord, leading to possible ischemia. The most common age group is 12 to 18 years old.

- *Causes:* It is not always known, but it can be attributed to an anatomic abnormality known as the "bell clapper deformity." This deformity allows the cords to twist more easily.
- *Signs and symptoms:* Acute, sudden, severe testicular pain radiating to groin or abdomen; NV; and elevated/swollen/tender testes.
- *Interventions:* Anticipate orders for IV crystalloid fluids and analgesics, ice packs, and testicular ultrasound; prepare for manual reduction of the torsion, or prepare for surgery as indicated.

Notes: _____

Penile Fracture

Penile fracture is an acute rupture in the membrane (tunica albuginea) that surrounds the corpora cavernosa.

- *Causes:* Trauma or abrupt bending of the erect penis commonly associated with aggressive sexual intercourse or masturbation.
- *Signs and symptoms:* The patient may report hearing a cracking or popping sound upon injury, immediately followed by pain, flaccidity, hematoma, swelling, deformity, and dark bruising of the penis. Other symptoms may include hematuria, blood noted at the urethral meatus, and inability to void.
- *Interventions:* Anticipate orders to administer pain medications, insert IV access, obtain urinalysis if possible, contact emergent consulting urologist, and give patient nothing by mouth and *no* urethral catheterizations. Prepare for retrograde urethrogram, and surgical intervention with transfer to the operating room.

Notes: _____

Urinary Retention

Urinary retention (ischuria) is the inability to void or to fully empty the bladder.

- *Causes:* Enlarged prostate, constipation, infection, nerve dysfunction, urethral obstruction or strictures, kidney stones, blood clots, and some medications such as opioids, amphetamines, anticholinergics, antidepressants, and COX-2 inhibitors.
- *Signs and symptoms:* Unable to void or "only a little comes out"; bladder "feels full" or is distended; lower mid-abdominal pain; and patient may appear anxious.
- *Interventions:* To properly treat urinary retention, one must first find the cause by obtaining an accurate urological history and assessment. Anticipate orders to obtain urology consult, and insert Foley catheter. If resistance is met upon Foley catheter insertion, do not force; reattempt with a smaller or specialty Foley catheter per order. Once inserted, the patient typically finds instant relief. To avoid bladder spasms, clamp the Foley after the first 1,000 mL empties into the Foley bag.

Notes: _____

Genital Warts

Genital warts (condylomata acuminate) is a viral sexually transmitted infection. The virus responsible is the human papilloma virus (HPV). It is estimated that about 50% of sexually active males and females will acquire HPV in their lifetime.

- *Causes:* Sexual contact with an infected partner.
- *Signs and symptoms:* Painless single or multipapular-type rash in various shapes such as plaque or cauliflower-like appearance to the genital areas. Areas affected may include perianal, vulva, penis, perineum, and cervix. The oral pharynx or larynx may also be affected. Warts may spontaneously increase or decrease without treatment.
- *Interventions:* Because it is a viral infection, there is no cure. Treatments may include laser therapy, surgical excision, and/or cryotherapy. The treatment goal is to remove symptomatic warts to induce more "wart-free" periods. Although there is no cure, we can educate our patients on prevention. The Gardasil vaccine is now available to prevent cervical cancer and other diseases associated with HPV.

Notes: _____

Priapism

Priapism is a prolonged painful penile erection lasting longer than 4 to 6 hours.

- *Common causes:* Spinal cord injury, leukemia, sickle cell disease, psychotropic drugs, multiple sclerosis, prolonged sexual stimulation, penile tumor, urethral tumor, anticoagulant therapy, and impotence treatments.
- *Signs and symptoms:* Prolonged painful penile erection for more than 4 to 6 hours.
- *Treatments:* Anticipate treatment of underlying causes by provider that may include observation of patient, ice packs, penile or groin pressure, intracavernous injections (with drugs such as epinephrine, norepinephrine, and ephedrine), needle aspiration, or surgery.

Notes: _____

Question: How do you treat a 19-year-old male who arrives at the ED stating that his penis is stuck in his pants zipper?
Answer: *Cut it off. Not the penis, the zipper! Control bleeding and provide ice packs.*

SUMMARY

Although most genitourinary emergencies can be treated with medications, some require immediate interventions. Remember that renal infections, obstructions, or poor perfusion can lead to renal failure; early intervention is key. You should now understand some of the most frequent problems that bring patients to the ED and how to treat them promptly and effectively.

11

Geriatric Emergencies

As the baby boomer generation ages, we can anticipate an even higher volume of emergency department (ED) patients. **The normal physiological changes of the aging process leave patients more vulnerable to illness, injuries, and complications.** Several important body systems also slow down. Many geriatric patients have decreased renal function, decreased circulation, thinner skin, weaker bones, less muscle mass, decreased hearing, decreased gastric motility, brain atrophy, and visual impairments. It is always important to take these age-related changes into consideration when caring for older patients. As you review this chapter, you will learn some of the most common geriatric emergencies and how to handle them.

During this part of your orientation, locate and become familiar with:

- Assistive walking devices (e.g., canes and walkers)
- Adult protective services and social services
- Facility policy for reporting elder abuse
- Denture containers
- Fall risk assessments and precautions

DIAGNOSES

Fast Facts in a Nutshell

- Normal physiological changes leave older patients more vulnerable to illness, injuries, and complications.
- Geriatric patients may have decreased renal function, decreased circulation, thinner skin, weaker bones, decreased hearing, decreased gastric motility, brain atrophy, poor thermoregulation, and visual impairments.
- Blood urea nitrogen and creatinine levels naturally increase with age.

Elder Abuse

Elder abuse can take several different forms, including physical, sexual, financial, and psychological; it can also include neglect. Abuse is physical harm, pain, or mental anguish; neglect is the failure to provide services or goods needed to prevent physical harm and mental anguish. Elder abuse is an international problem that can be difficult to detect. Females are more commonly abused than males. **You must report all suspected abuse!**

- *Causes:* Not always known. Elder abuse can occur in any socioeconomic group. Lack of resources and stressed or burned-out caregivers can contribute to the problem.
- *Signs and symptoms:* Conflicting stories describing how an injury occurred; patient not given an opportunity to speak; time lapse between injury and presentation to the ED; disinterested caregiver; history of similar injuries; hand marks; bite marks; multiple bruises; multiple fractures in various healing stages; altered ambulation from sexual assault; malnourishment; dehydration; poor hygiene; withdrawal; and agitation.
- *Interventions:* Treat injuries and illness; *accurately document* and photograph injuries or neglect per policy; ascertain whether report needs to be filed; notify social services as soon as possible; obtain supportive services through community referrals; consider hospitalization to ensure patient safety; and refer to adult protective services.

Notes: _____

Falls

Many geriatric injuries or illnesses are associated with falls. Complications often include soft tissue injuries, hip fractures, Colles' fracture (wrist), subdural hematoma, and hot-water burns from falls in the bathtub. First, assess the reason for the fall. Were there any symptoms prior to the fall (e.g., dizziness, chest pain, and loss of consciousness)? What was the activity during the fall? The location? Are there any witnesses? Any history of falls or alcohol intake? Finally, assess whether the patient fell at ground level. If not, how many feet did the patient fall?

- *Causes:* Can be attributed to impaired vision, sensation, neuro-circulatory system, gait, and balance.
- *Signs and symptoms:* Depend on the fall and injuries.
- *Interventions:* Give nothing by mouth; consider cervical injury and immobilization (rest, ice, splint, and elevate injury); clean and apply sterile dressing to wounds; assess pain; administer pain medications as ordered; arrange neurological exams; monitor extremity movement; and check circulation. Prepare for diagnostic studies. Educate patient and family on fall prevention.

Notes: _____

Syncope

Syncope is transient loss of consciousness with a spontaneous recovery.

- *Causes:* Identifying the cause may prove to be more valuable than treating the sustained injuries. Assess patient's activity just before the syncopal event.
  - Temporary, abrupt decrease in cardiac output due to aortic stenosis, mitral valve disease, cardiomyopathy, dysrhythmias, and sick sinus syndrome.
  - Volume depletion due to hemorrhage/anemia, diuresis, dehydration, and third-space fluid shift.
  - Hypersensitive carotid sinus due to neck turning, constrictive collars, and drugs (digitalis, propranolol hydrochloride, and alpha-methyldopa).
  - Vasovagal response with hypotension due to cough, defecation, or urination.
  - Hypoglycemia or hypoxia.

- *Signs and symptoms:* Dizziness; chest pain; dyspnea; weakness; confusion; loss of consciousness; witnesses to the fall; and previous history.
- *Interventions:* Anticipate orders to obtain serum glucose and complete basic metabolic panel; administer oxygen through nasal cannula; check pulse oxygen; perform electrocardiogram and CT scan.
  - If due to adult hypoglycemia, treat intravenously with dextrose 50% injection (D50; 1 amp) or give oral or intramuscular injection of glucose. Then feed patient once he or she is alert and oriented to person, place, and time.

Notes: _____

Dehydration

Dehydration is a lack of required serum fluid levels. Elderly patients are more prone to dehydration because of normal physiological changes that occur with aging.

- *Causes:* Altered sense of thirst; decrease in total body fluid; decreased kidney function; and decreased effectiveness of antidiuretic hormone, which helps conserve water.
- *Signs and symptoms:* Confusion; seizure; dry oral mucosa; dry skin; sunken eyes; lethargy; headache; constipation; hyperthermia; weak rapid pulse; orthostatic hypotension; altered respiration; concentrated urine; and decreased urine output.
- *Interventions:* Anticipate orders to administer fluids intravenously or by mouth, assess mental status, check vital signs, and measure intake and output. Diagnostic studies may include metabolic panel, hematocrit, blood urea nitrogen, and complete blood count (CBC).

Notes: _____

Dementia

Also known as "major neurocognitive disorder," dementia is commonly mistaken for normal age-related cognitive changes. However, with dementia, the onset is more severe with an abrupt onset.

- *Causes:* Not always known, but may be attributed to electrolyte imbalance, dehydration, infection, and stroke. This assessment requires input from caregivers to determine the patient's normal cognitive baseline.

- *Signs and symptoms:* Alert with impaired orientation; impaired recent memory; impoverished thinking; difficulty finding words; confused speech; and poor sleep.
- *Interventions:* Provide a safe environment; put bed in low, locked position; monitor patient closely (place close to nurses' station); and assess for any new causes of confusion. Anticipate orders for intravenous (IV) access, IV fluids, CBC with differential, metabolic panel, urinalysis, toxicology screen, chest x-ray, head CT, and if possible have family or sitter available at the bedside to redirect or reorient patient.
  - Common cause of confusion in elderly is *pneumonia* or *urinary tract infection.*

Notes: _____

Alzheimer's Disease

Alzheimer's disease affects one in eight people older than 65 years of age. It is a chronic, progressive, irreversible, degenerative dementia that has no preventive measures or cure.

- *Causes:* Unknown with focus studies on loss of synapses in the brain.
- *Signs and symptoms:* Forgetfulness; memory loss; paranoia; delusions; irritability; depression; aphasia; apraxia; and history of progressive deteriorating mental functioning.
- *Interventions:* Prevent patient from injuring self or others; provide supervised safe environment with minimal stimulation; give short explanations and simple instructions; involve support-ive services (social services); and provide health care resources and community referrals.

Notes: _____

Pneumonia

Pneumonia is a bacterial, viral, or fungal infection below the bronchi resulting in inflammation of lung parenchyma.

- *Causes:* Bacterial, viral, or fungal lung infection. Contributing factors include a weak immune system; general debilitated condition; decreased mobility; chronic cardiac disease; chronic pulmonary disease; weak cough reflex; aspiration; late diagnosis; and diabetes.

- *Signs and symptoms:* Confusion; change in normal activity; anorexia; tachypnea; dyspnea; fever or subnormal temperature; dehydration; productive or nonproductive cough; chills; weakness; chest pain; nausea and vomiting; abdominal distention; diaphoresis; cyanosis; and diminished lung sounds or crackles.
- *Interventions:* Anticipate orders for chest x-ray, CBC, blood cultures, and arterial blood gases. Start IV access, maintain bed rest, and give fluids intravenously; pulse oximeter monitoring, along with oxygen and antibiotics as ordered.

Notes: _____

Urosepsis

Urosepsis is an infection caused by urinary tract infection that is more common in women than in men. In general, urinary infections are the most common bacterial infections in the elderly. Urosepsis may lead to septic shock.

- *Causes:* Predisposing factors include an indwelling catheter and kidney stones.
- *Signs and symptoms:* Confusion; lethargy; altered mental status; tachycardia; tachypnea; fever or subnormal temperature; urinary frequency; urinary urgency; incontinence; nausea and vomiting; abdominal tenderness; and hypotension.
- *Interventions:* Anticipate orders to obtain urinalysis, administer fluids and antibiotics intravenously, and monitor urinary output. Prepare for possible admission.

Notes: _____

Question: What are the common causes associated with acute onset of altered mental status in elderly patients?
Answer: *Urosepsis and pneumonia.*

SUMMARY

You now have a better understanding of the diseases most commonly associated with elderly patients in the ED. Age-related physiological changes in elderly patients will affect their condition and can lead to complications. Be sure to assess and document these patients carefully. Obtain histories from them and their caregivers, when available. Caring for elderly patients can be a blessing. Often, they are more appreciative than younger patients.

12

Hematological Emergencies

Some hematological emergencies, such as anemia, sickle cell anemia, and hemophilia, are commonly seen in the emergency department (ED), while others, such as leukemia and lymphoma, are rarer. Regardless, an ED nurse should be able to help identify and anticipate appropriate interventions. Remember to treat pain according to the patient's report. Just because you cannot see the pain does not mean it is not there. For example, a patient with sickle cell pain may play a game on his or her phone to distract from the pain. Document both subjective and objective data. Take the time to review your hospital's blood transfusion procedure with your preceptor; often, your colleagues in the blood bank department can serve as an excellent resource.

During this part of your orientation, locate and become familiar with:

- Blood transfusion supplies: Blood tubing, forms and documentation, and hospital protocol
- Warming devices
- Neutropenic precautions
- Medications to know: Morphine, hydromorphone (Dilaudid), ketorolac (Toradol), diphenhydramine (Benadryl), ondansetron (Zofran), promethazine (Phenergan), and factor VIII and IX replacement therapy

ANEMIA

Anemia, simply put, is a lack of oxygen-carrying red blood cells (RBCs) or hemoglobin. It can be mild or severe, acute or chronic. It is characterized by a low hemoglobin and hematocrit (H & H) level. In men, the normal hemoglobin level is less than 13.5% and the hematocrit level is less than 39 g/dL. In women, the normal hemoglobin level is less than 12% and the hematocrit is less than 36 g/dL.

- *Causes:* Blood loss due to trauma or gastrointestinal (GI) bleeding, destruction of RBCs, or inadequate RBC production. Common types of anemia include iron deficiency, vitamin deficiency, aplastic, hemolytic, sickle cell, thalassemia, and malarial. In addition, chronic inflammatory diseases such as cancer, HIV, kidney and Crohn's disease, and certain toxins or venoms can interfere with RBC production. It is not uncommon for patients older than 65 to have chronic mild anemia.
- *Signs and symptoms:* Weakness; fatigue; dizziness; headache; pallor; dyspnea; dysrhythmias; chest pain; and cool extremities.
- *Interventions:* Assess and treat underlying causes based on type of anemia. Anticipate orders to provide oxygen, control and reassess any hemorrhaging, establish large-bore intravenous (IV) access, monitor vital signs, monitor oximetry or wave form capnography, apply warming measure, and avoid nonsteroidal anti-inflammatory drugs (NSAIDs) if cause is bleeding. Anticipate orders to collect a complete blood count (CBC) with differential, coagulation studies, and type and crossmatch. Prepare for possible blood transfusion.

Notes: _____

Fast Facts in a Nutshell

Quickly determine pallor regardless of skin type by assessing the palms of the patient's hands in addition to the inside lower eyelids and oral mucosa. Document a thorough circulatory assessment, including vital signs, capnometry, oximetry, color, temperature, and capillary refill of extremities before and after interventions to determine effectiveness.

SICKLE CELL ANEMIA

Sickle cell anemia is an inherited hemolytic form of anemia. The RBCs contain too much hemoglobin S causing the RBC to take on a sickle or crescent-like shape instead of a normal tubular or jelly doughnut-like shape. Sickle-shaped blood cells tend to clump together in smaller or constricted vessels causing blockage or vaso-occlusive crisis. Similar to an acute myocardial infarction (AMI), the vessel obstruction can lead to poor tissue perfusion and eventually necrosis of surrounding tissue. Complications may include stroke, acute chest syndrome, organ and joint damage, aplastic crisis, splenic sequestration, priapism, pulmonary hypertension, pulmonary embolism, renal failure, and retinal occlusion resulting in blindness.

- *Causes:* Inheriting two sickle cell genes from one's parents. According to the Centers for Disease Control and Prevention (CDC), sickle cell anemia affects millions of people around the world. Primarily it affects Black or African Americans, but is also found in Hispanic, Arabic, Indian, and Mediterranean races. Although it is extremely risky, stem cell or bone marrow transplants offer a possible hope for a future cure.
- *Signs and symptoms:* Typically, patients present with pain, but may also present with weakness, fatigue, dizziness, headache, pallor, dyspnea, dysrhythmias, chest pain, joint pain, delayed growth, fever, infections, and swollen or cool extremities.
- *Interventions:* Apply warming measures, pulse oximetry or waveform capnography, cardiac monitor, and supplemental oxygen if pulse oximetry reading is less than 92% to 94%. Anticipate orders for frequent vital signs, IV access, high-dose IV or subcutaneous opioids, analgesics, antiemetics, NSAIDs, and Benadryl (diphenhydramine). If patient is hypovolemic, isotonic crystalloid or hypotonic IV fluids may be ordered. It is recommended that analgesics be administered within 30 to 60 minutes of arrival. Blood transfusions may be ordered if the patient is in critical condition. Diagnostic tests may include CBC with differential, metabolic panel, reticulocyte count, and liver function test. Most sickle cell patients manage their disease proactively with their hematologists or primary care physicians. However, there will be a few who routinely use the ED to manage their care. A hospital or ED social worker may be able to assist

connecting the patient with better community sickle cell resources and follow-up care upon discharge.

Notes: _____

True or False: Diagnostic tests can be used to validate the pain in a sickle cell patient.
Answer: *False, patient report of severity should guide management of pain.*

Question: Decades ago, sickle cell anemia was considered a childhood illness as many did not survive to see adulthood. Today the average life expectancy is:
a. 30
b. 40
c. 50
d. 60
Answer: *b is correct.*

DISSEMINATED INTRAVASCULAR COAGULATION

Disseminated intravascular coagulation typically results from a primary complication that triggers a massive coagulation pathway in the body. As a result, thrombocytopenia, fibrinolysis, and thrombosis may occur leading to systemic bleeding and micro-coagulation.

- *Causes:* A primary infection or inflammatory process; trauma; burns; shock; obstetric emergencies; sepsis; snake bite; heat stroke; or cancer.

- *Signs and symptoms:* Uncontrolled bleeding; petechial rash; purpura rash; oozing blood from venipuncture sites; hypoxia; and organ necrosis.
- *Interventions:* Anticipate orders to control any external hemorrhage, give oxygen, treat primary causes, obtain multiple large-bore IV accesses, and administer fresh frozen plasma (FFP), platelets, and cryoprecipitate with fibrinogen as ordered.

Notes: _____

HEMOPHILIA

Hemophilia is a rare congenital bleeding disorder related to poor clotting. It occurs primarily in males.

- *Causes:* Genetic defect of clotting factor IIIV (type A) or clotting factor IX (type B or Christmas disease). This particular genetic defect is passed down from mother to son. Genetic researchers continue to search for a cure.
- *Signs and symptoms:* Excessive internal or external bleeding; bruising; prolonged nasal bleeding; hematuria; tarry stools; coffee ground emesis; painful joint swelling; or signs of increased cranial pressure (ICP) if bleeding is present in the brain.
- *Interventions:* Triage a high risk priority patient (ESI level 2). Anticipate orders to obtain IV access and immediate administration of clotting factor IIIV or IX replacement IV as indicated. Other orders may include: desmopressin acetate (DDAVP) administration for minor bleeding, joint elevation; ice; and immobilization, hematologist consult, and topical thrombin for nose bleeds. Diagnostic tests should not delay IV clotting factor replacement but may include CTs, x-rays, CBC, prothrombin time (PT), partial thromboplastin time (PTT), and factor levels. Most parents are a helpful resource as their children receive infusions weekly or routinely as preventative maintenance; they may even carry their own factor replacement with them to the ED.

Notes: _____

Intramuscular (IM) injections and repeated venipunctures in a hemophiliac patient should be avoided, as they may result in large painful hematomas. When obtaining labs and IV access, consider:

- Utilizing an experienced IV therapist
- Tying the tourniquet loosely to avoid bruising
- Using smaller gauge needle if patient is hemodynamically stable
- Applying direct pressure for 3 to 5 minutes afterward

LEUKEMIA

Leukemia is a cancer of the blood, blood-producing organs, and bone marrow.

- *Causes:* Damaged DNA or mutated bone marrow cells lead to an over production of blast cells, the precursors to WBCs. These cancerous blast cells never develop into healthy blood cells affecting platelet, RBC, and WBC production. There are several types of leukemia. The cause of this mutation is unknown but risk factors may include previous exposure to chemotherapy or radiation, chemical exposures such as benzene, family history of leukemia, smoking, and Down syndrome.
- *Signs and symptoms:* May include bruising; pallor; dyspnea; petechial or purpura rash; epistaxis; weakness; loss of appetite; weight loss; fever; frequent opportunistic infections; joint pain; swollen lymph nodes; splenomegaly; and hepatomegaly.
- *Interventions:* Anticipate orders to obtain CBC with differential, coagulation studies, chemistry, CT, x-rays, lumbar puncture, and large-bore IV access. Possible blood transfusion, antibiotics, hematologist or oncologist consult, and neutropenic precautions may also be ordered. Definitive diagnosis may be made following a bone marrow biopsy.

Notes: _____

Question: Which nursing action is of greatest priority for a patient with bone pain related to leukemia?
a. Administer pain medication
b. Place patient in a private room
c. Administer oxygen
d. Discuss advance directives
Answer: *b is correct.*

Leukemia patients are highly susceptible to infection; a nosocomial infection could prove deadly. Place patient on reverse isolation upon arrival.

LYMPHOMA

Lymphoma is a rare cancer of the lymphatic system.

- *Causes:* Unknown but risk factors may include certain types of chemical, viral, or bacterial exposures. Can be further classified into Hodgkin's and non-Hodgkin's lymphoma. Patients may present to the ED with obstructions and immunosuppression complications.
- *Signs and symptoms:* Painless swollen lymph nodes; abdominal pain or swelling; chest pain; cough; dyspnea; fatigue; fever; night sweats; and weight loss. Complications may include swelling of upper airway, hypercalcemia, pericardial effusion with tamponade, spinal cord syndrome, and superior vena cava syndrome.
- *Interventions:* Treat airway, breathing, and circulation (ABCs) first, and anticipate orders for CBC with differential, coagulation studies, erythrocyte sedimentation rate, liver functions, blood urea nitrogen (BUN), creatinine, lumbar puncture (LP) if neurological system is affected, x-rays, CTs or MRIs of affected areas, and neutropenic precautions if patient is receiving chemotherapy or radiation. An endocrine or oncologist referral may be obtained to confirm diagnosis with lymph node or bone marrow biopsy.

Notes: _____

SUMMARY

Due to advances in treatment options, patients today are surviving and living longer with hematological diseases. Anemia, sickle cell crisis, and hemophilia are more commonly seen in the ED than other hematological emergencies. Sickle cell pain interventions should be initiated ideally within 30 to 60 minutes of arrival. Be sure to review your hospital's process for type and crossmatch and blood transfusions. Ensure proper documents are completed such as blood consent, blood request, and transfusion assessments.

13

Infectious Disease Emergencies

Infectious diseases are common emergencies that must not be taken lightly. Usually, it is the triage nurse who is first exposed to the unknown case of tuberculosis or meningitis. Most infectious disease patients do not know what is wrong with them when they come to the emergency department (ED). Your facility should have a triage screening to alert the staff for infectious disease risks. If the triage screening is positive, you must follow your facilities protocol; this usually requires some sort of mask and isolation. The best advice I can give you is to assess your patients **carefully** and **wash your hands, wash your hands, wash your hands!** Most ED nurses frequently catch more colds and flus in their first year, so be careful. This chapter educates you on the different types of infectious diseases and how to handle them.

During this part of your orientation, locate and become familiar with:

- Wound cultures
- Lumbar puncture supplies, specimens, and procedures
- Contact, respiratory, and reverse isolation policies
- Personal protective equipment
- Incision and drainage supplies
- Triage screening for infectious diseases
- Policy for reporting disease to infection control personnel

■ Always practice universal/standard precautions.

DIAGNOSES

Clostridium difficile Infection (*C. diff*)

C. diff is a bacterial infection of the colon that affects more than half a million people annually and is becoming more difficult to treat. It is spread via contaminated feces or unwashed hands, and ingested orally. Its spores can survive for weeks to months.

■ *Causes:* Exposure to spore-producing *C. diff* bacteria or recent use of antibiotics. In the past, elderly age and exposure in health care facilities posed increased risks. Today, community-acquired *C. diff* is becoming more prevalent.
■ *Signs and symptoms:* Severe frequent liquid diarrhea, abdominal pain and cramping, nausea, fever, and abdominal distention. Diarrhea containing *C. diff* has a distinct foul odor; many experienced nurses can walk into a room and identify *C. diff* based solely on smell. I have known patients suffering from *C. diff* who constantly leaked liquid diarrhea. After continual changing of disposable pads, diapers, and bed linen, a rectal tube was ordered.
■ *Interventions:* Place patient on enteric contact precautions and implement strict handwashing. Anticipate orders for intravenous (IV) fluids, antiemetics, complete blood count with differential, basic metabolic panel, and stool culture. Mild cases may be treated with probiotics; severe cases may require antibiotics and admission.

Notes: _____

Meningitis

Meningitis is a bacterial, viral, or fungal infection of the meninges, which are membrane coverings of the brain.

- *Causes:* It usually starts as a sinus infection that spreads to the meninges.
- *Signs and symptoms:* "The worst headache of my life"; stiff neck (nuchal rigidity); lethargy; seizures; vomiting; confusion; and high fever. Infants may be febrile; irritable; crying; have bulging fontanels; nonblanching rash (purpura); vomiting; and have a poor appetite.
    - Kernig's sign is indicative of meningitis (low back/posterior thigh pain with hip flexion and gradual knee extension).
- *Interventions:* Place patient on droplet precautions during triage until test results return negative. Anticipate following orders: administer antipyretics; document frequent vital signs and neurological assessments; prepare a complete blood count, blood cultures, metabolic panel, and coagulation studies; set up for lumbar puncture; and administer IV fluids and medications (mannitol, steroids, antibiotics, vasopressors and/or inotropes).
    - Bacterial meningitis reveals an elevated white blood cell count greater than 1,000 cells/mm^3 and low glucose in the cerebrospinal fluid (CSF). It is more serious and requires antibiotics such as rifampin. Teach the patient that rifampin is an antibiotic that turns urine and tears orange.
    - Viral meningitis reveals mildly elevated white blood cell count of 100 to 1,000 cells/mm^3 or greater and normal glucose in the CSF. It may require antiviral medication, but usually resolves on its own.

Notes: _____

Fast Facts in a Nutshell

Providers will tell you positioning is key for obtaining a good lumbar puncture. For better positioning during a sitting lumbar puncture, place a step stool under the patient's feet. This brings the knees closer to the chest.

- Ensure each CSF collection tube is labeled correctly
    - Tube 1—glucose and protein
    - Tube 2—cell count with differential
    - Tube 3—Gram stain culture
    - Tube 4—repeat cell count with differential or other studies

HIV/AIDS

The human immunodeficiency virus (HIV) is a virus that attacks the immune system, allowing other pathogens to invade the body. Acquired immunodeficiency syndrome (AIDS) is a chronic, life-threatening condition caused by HIV. In the ED, we are to treat the acute complication of AIDS.

- *Causes:* Contamination by HIV through blood or body fluid exchange.
- *Signs and symptoms:* Early manifestations are similar to cold and flu symptoms. Later symptoms include weight loss; fever; shortness of breath; mouth ulcers; cough; sores that would not heal; and swollen lymph nodes.
  - Abnormally low CD4 lymphocyte count may be present.
  - Common opportunistic infections include bacterial pneumonia; tuberculosis; herpes; human papillomavirus; thrush; cryptococcal meningitis; *Pneumocystis carinii* pneumonia; Kaposi's sarcoma; and non-Hodgkin's lymphoma.
- *Interventions:* Anticipate orders to treat opportunistic infections, maintain appropriate isolation depending on complications, monitor vital signs, administer acetaminophen for fever, prepare a complete blood count, perform HIV testing (enzyme-linked immunosorbent assay and Western blot tests) if unknown case, request chest x-ray, culture wounds, and obtain IV access.

Notes: _____

Fast Facts in a Nutshell

We do not perform routine HIV testing in the ED because we cannot provide follow-up care. Your local health department can provide routine HIV testing.

Patients taking corticosteroids will have an elevated white blood cell count.

Hepatitis

Hepatitis is an inflammation or infection of the liver.

- *Causes:* Alcohol abuse; overdose of medications; IV drug abuse; autoimmune disorders; contaminated food or water; and presence of hepatitis A, B, C, D, or E virus.
  - *Hepatitis A:* Contracted via fecal oral route; children are typically asymptomatic.
  - *Hepatitis B:* Contracted via blood or body fluids.
  - *Hepatitis C:* Contracted via blood or body fluid, commonly in IV drug abusers.
  - *Hepatitis D:* Contracted via blood or body fluids; requires coinfection of hepatitis B.
  - *Hepatitis E:* Contracted via fecal oral route with higher mortality rate than hepatitis A.
- *Signs and symptoms:* May be asymptomatic or have ascites; chills; fever; malaise; jaundice; elevated liver enzymes; right upper quadrant abdominal pain; dark urine; anorexia; diarrhea or constipation; and nausea and vomiting. The patient often looks like Big Bird—yellow all over with a big round belly.
- *Interventions:* Anticipate orders to medicate for pain, nausea, and vomiting; administer vaccine or immunoglobulin; complete a basic metabolic panel; perform a liver function test and coagulation studies; check for abnormal bleeding; and educate the patient to stop any alcohol consumption or use of acetaminophen.

Notes: _____

Cellulitis/Abscess/MRSA

Abscesses are pockets of skin infection that look like giant pimples ranging in size from a marble to a golf ball or larger. Diabetic patients are at higher risk for cellulitis and poor healing.

- *Causes:* Most abscesses are caused from methicillin-resistant *Staphylococcus aureus* (MRSA). Others may come from other types of bacteria, clogged hair follicles, or clogged pores.
- *Signs and symptoms:* Pain; redness and warmth to affected area; proximal red streaks; pus; and/or fever.
- *Interventions:* Anticipate orders to maintain contact isolation, prepare patient for possible incision and drainage of abscess; if

appropriate, pack the wound, bandage the wound, and administer antibiotics and warm compresses.

■ Educate the patient on how to prevent the spread of MRSA (wash hands and bleach everything). MRSA lives dormant under fingernails and in nostrils. This is why your mom said not to pick your nose! Providers may prescribe antibiotic ointment to apply inside nostrils.

Notes: _____

Febrile Neutropenia

A febrile neutropenic patient is immunocompromised with a fever or a possible infection.

■ *Causes:* These are usually patients receiving chemotherapy. For them, a low-grade fever, say 99.9°F, is of concern because their immune systems are too weak to handle it.
■ *Signs and symptoms:* Fever and possibly cold- or flu-like symptoms.
■ *Interventions:* Reverse isolation with neutropenic precautions. During triage or in waiting room, provide patient with a mask for his or her own protection until placed in isolation room. Monitor vital signs; anticipate orders to administer acetaminophen or ibuprofen (for fever) and antibiotics, prepare a complete blood count, obtain an IV access, and prepare for possible admission.

Notes: _____

Tick-Borne Illnesses

These are infectious diseases caused by ticks.

Lyme disease: A *Borrelia burgdorferi* bacterial infection (see Figure 13.1).

■ *Causes:* Usually spread by deer ticks.
■ *Signs and symptoms:* Vary by individual, but commonly include a "bull's-eye" rash at site of tick bite and flu-like symptoms (fever, chills, joint pain, fatigue, and swollen lymph nodes). Neurological problems may be a late sign and include Bell's palsy, dizziness, nerve pain, and extremity numbness.
■ *Interventions:* Remove all ticks and administer antibiotics (e.g., doxycycline or amoxicillin) as ordered.

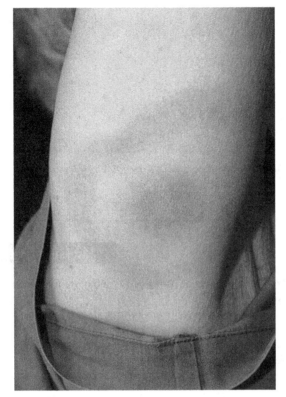

Figure 13.1 Bull's-eye rash of Lyme disease.

Notes: _____

Rocky Mountain spotted fever: A bacterial infection transmitted by ticks (see Figure 13.2).

- *Causes:* Bite from tick contaminated with *Rickettsia rickettsii* bacteria.
- *Signs and symptoms:* High fever; tick bite 2 to 14 days earlier; poor appetite; headache; body aches; nausea and vomiting; abdominal pain; fatigue; and red spotted rash in 90% of cases.
- *Interventions:* Anticipate orders to remove all ticks; obtain complete blood count, metabolic panel, liver enzymes, and coagulation studies; and administer antibiotics (e.g., doxycycline) as ordered.

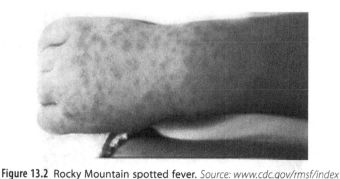

Figure 13.2 Rocky Mountain spotted fever. *Source: www.cdc.gov/rmsf/index .html*

Notes: _____

Fast Facts in a Nutshell

- For easy tick removal, use tweezers and grasp the head portion (see Figure 13.3).
- Pull steadily and evenly from its head.
- If any mouth pieces remain, use tweezers to remove them.
- Thoroughly cleanse the tick bite area with soap and water, antiseptic solution, or rubbing alcohol.
- Dispose by flushing down the toilet.

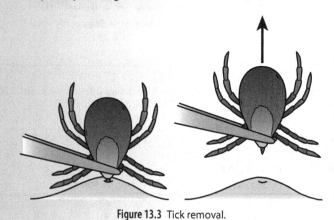

Figure 13.3 Tick removal.

Notes: _____

Toxic Shock Syndrome

Toxic shock syndrome is a life-threatening *S. aureus* or group A beta-hemolytic strep bacterial infection.

- *Causes:* May occur with recent surgery, burns, or open wounds and the use of tampons vaginally or nasally. The toxins released from these two bacteria can cause the patient to go into septic shock *very rapidly*—sometimes right before your eyes.
- *Signs and symptoms:* Similar to septic shock but with faster onset. Includes sudden high fever; hypotension; headache; confusion; tachycardia; nausea, vomiting, and diarrhea; sunburn-like rash with desquamation (skin peeling); fatigue; and seizures.
- *Interventions:* You must work rapidly. Place patient on contact isolation. Monitor vital signs; anticipate orders to insert a large-bore IV access for administration of IV isotonic fluid bolus and, as soon as possible, antibiotics; place in modified Trendelenburg position for hypotension; prepare a complete blood count; take blood cultures; remove any foreign body in any body cavity and get a wound culture (if source is vaginal, prepare for pelvic exam with cultures); give norepinephrine or dopamine for hypotension, and antipyretics; and prepare for possible intensive care unit admission.
  - If the patient is stable, try to obtain blood cultures before giving antibiotics. If unstable, give the antibiotics now!

Notes: _____

Tuberculosis

In its *active phase,* tuberculosis is a life-threatening bacterial infection that commonly attacks the lungs but can attack other organs as well.

- *Causes:* Mycobacterium tuberculosis is spread via droplet, so negative pressure respiratory isolation is necessary. In its dormant stage, tuberculosis is not contagious, and patient is asymptomatic.
- *Signs and symptoms:* The patient can be asymptomatic or have a cough lasting several weeks; coughing up blood; fever; night sweats; and fatigue.
- *Interventions:* Screen patients for tuberculosis in triage and provide mask to suspected patients. Then place the patient in

room on respiratory isolation. Anticipate orders to obtain IV access, request a chest x-ray, obtain a complete blood count, administer antibiotics (e.g., isoniazid and rifampin), and prepare for possible admission. Instruct family members and caregivers to get tuberculosis testing. Be sure to document the time droplet negative pressure respiratory isolation was initiated and if mask was provided in triage or waiting room.

Notes: _____

Question: What drug besides phenazopyridine (Pyridium) makes your urine orange?
Answer: *Rifampin.*

To remember drugs used to treat tuberculosis, just remember RIPE—**R**ifampin, **I**soniazid, **P**yrazinamide, and **E**thambutol.

SUMMARY

Most EDs do not allow new graduate nurses to triage until proper training and experience are achieved. This is partly because the triage nurses are the front line when it comes to exposure to infectious diseases. Therefore, it is crucial to thoroughly screen all patients who come through triage for infectious diseases. If an infectious disease is suspected, proper isolation must be implemented. Make sure you become familiar with your facility's isolation protocols and equipment and know how to use it. This information may seem a bit scary at first, but look around you. There are ED nurses who have been doing this for decades! The key is good handwashing, universal precautions, triage screening, and proper isolation.

14

Mental Health Emergencies

I have to admit, mental health emergencies may not be everyone's favorite topic. We can all empathize; everyone experiences anxiety, stress, anger, and depression in their lives, but some people become suicidal, violent, or psychotic. Mental health patients may be difficult to treat at times, particularly when they engage in disruptive behavior. At times, security, antianxiety medication, seclusion, and restraints may be necessary for short periods of time to maintain patient safety. However, restraints should be a last resort after the least restrictive measures have been attempted. Restraint legal documentation requirements can be intense and vary according to the purpose (medical/nonviolent vs. violent/behavior). Take the time to learn the various restraint documentation requirements during orientation. Be aware that state suicide intent documentation does not always necessitate restraints and vice versa. **Your priority must always be to maintain safety for yourself, your staff members, your patient, and other patients.** However, you will find that most mental health patients respond better if you listen, respect their personal space, and educate them on all procedures clearly and early on.

During this part of your orientation, locate and become familiar with:

- Your state's and facility's seclusion-and-restraint policies
- Restraint-and-seclusion forms
- Legal suicidal intent documents
- Transfer policies to mental health facilities

(continued)

- Local mental health counselors and facilities
- Your facility's security and its codes
- Medications to know: Lorazepam (Ativan), haloperidol (Haldol), and ziprasidone (Geodon)

DIAGNOSES

Anxiety

Anxiety is a vague feeling of apprehension, tension, and uneasiness that can be divided into four levels: mild, moderate, severe, and panic.

- *Causes:* Usually some sort of stressor, but it varies with the individual and his or her circumstances.
- *Signs and symptoms by level:*
  - *Mild:* Minimal muscle tension; normal vital signs; constricted normal pupils; random controlled thoughts; and appearance of calm.
  - *Moderate:* Normal to slightly elevated vital signs; tension; excited behavior; alertness; optimum state for problem solving and learning; attentive; and energized.
  - *Severe:* Flight-or-fight response; tachycardia; tachypnea; hypertension; diaphoretic; urinary urgency; diarrhea; dry mouth; dilated pupils; difficulty in problem solving; feel overwhelmed; and decreased appetite.
  - *Panic:* Faint feeling or syncope from sympathetic nervous system release; pallor; hyperventilation; hypertension; pain; weakness; lack of coordination; choking or gasping sensation; chest pressure or lump in throat; helplessness; may become angry/combative/withdrawn, tearful; and shortness of breath.
- *Interventions:* Maintain calm and private environment; reduce stimulation; stay with the patient or have a support person stay; use simple repetitive communication; encourage verbalization of feelings; administer antianxiety/analgesic medications; evaluate effectiveness of medications; and teach relaxation/breathing techniques.

Notes: _____

Posttraumatic Stress Disorder

The disorder is a reaction to overwhelmingly traumatic events.

- *Causes:* A traumatic or overwhelming event such as military combat, rape, and natural or man-made disaster.
- *Signs and symptoms:* Signs of anxiety, hyperarousal, or stress; recurring dreams or flashbacks, which may be accompanied by dissociative reactions; explosive anger; increased substance abuse; sleep disturbances; difficulty concentrating; avoidance of activities surrounding the event; and feelings of guilt.
- *Interventions:* Assess suicidal/homicidal ideations; assess anxiety levels; provide therapeutic listening; avoid judgment; and provide referrals for group or individual counseling.

Notes: _____

Depression

Depression is a state of sadness or hopelessness that affects one mentally and physically. Short periods of depression following a specific event, such as divorce or death, are natural and resolve in time. However, clinical depression related to chemical or hormonal imbalances may require medication and therapy for a period of time or a lifetime.

- *Causes:* Vary by individual and circumstances. May be the natural result of a specific event, such as divorce or death, or may be more situational. If, however, it is the result of hormonal or chemical imbalances, the condition may require prolonged treatment.
- *Signs and symptoms:* Sad mood; lack of interest in or pleasure from activities; insomnia or hypersomnia; fatigue; feelings of guilt or worthlessness; inability to think or concentrate; inability to make decisions; anorexia; and suicidal ideation or attempt.
- *Interventions:* Assess suicide risk; discuss patient's emotional state; show interest and concern; and provide choices. Antidepressants are rarely administered in the emergency department (ED); they are not usually effective for the first week or two.

Notes: _____

- Monoamine oxidase inhibitors + alcohol = hypertensive crisis
- Monoamine oxidase inhibitors + foods that ferment (yogurt, cheeses, sour cream) = hypertensive crisis

Question: Why don't we typically discharge patients with antidepressant prescriptions?
Answer: *These patients need psychiatric follow-up and probably will not go if they are able to receive medications in the ED.*

Suicide

Suicide is an intentional self-inflicted death. Suicidal actions include suicidal thoughts, threats, gestures, and/or attempts.

- *Causes:* Vary by individual and circumstance. There are, however, common risk factors: male; age older than 65 years; Caucasian; substance/physical/sexual/mental/emotional abuse; depression; family history of or prior suicide attempt; terminal or chronic illness; psychosis; lives alone; recent change/loss in life; and low self-esteem.
- *Signs and symptoms:* Previous suicide attempts; verbal statements of suicidal thoughts; giving away favorite items; writing a will; depressed mood; isolated; and withdrawn.
- *Interventions:* Engage in one-to-one observation; remove any potentially dangerous objects (dress in a gown and remove personal belongings); encourage verbal expression of feelings/thoughts; promote hope; obtain labs as ordered for medical clearance; and obtain mental health evaluation. Assessment questions are listed as follows.
  - Are you having thoughts about ending your life?
  - If you had a way, would you try to take your own life?
  - Have you ever had specific thoughts or plans about ending your own life?
  - Have you set a time or place?
  - What are these plans?
  - Do you have access to _____ (this method)?

■ Have you done anything or made preparations to take your own life?

Notes: _____

SAD PERSONS Scale

Risk factors	Points
S—Sex	1 point if male; 0 if female
A—Age	1 point for age <20 or >44
D—Depression	1 point if present
P—Previous attempt	1 point if present
E—Ethanol abuse	1 point if present
R—Rational thinking loss	1 point if present
S—Social support lacking	1 point if present
O—Organized plan	1 point if plan is made and lethal
N—No spouse	1 if divorced, widowed, separated, or single
S—Sickness	1 if chronic, debilitating, and severe

Total points	Risk assessment
0–5	Low: May be safe for discharge
5–8	Moderate: Possible mental health consult required
8–10	High: Possible mental health admission

Fast Facts in a Nutshell

■ The 20-year-old suicidal male patient who describes to you in detail how he is going to commit suicide is the most dangerous.

Violent or Aggressive Behavior

This is behavior that has harmed or may result in harm to the patient or others.

■ *Causes:* Many factors can trigger aggressive behavior, including alcohol, drugs, or long waiting times in the ED.
■ *Signs and symptoms:* Loud/threatening speech; yelling profanities; bragging about past violence; demanding personality;

pacing; acting tense; clenching fists; slamming/pushing/throwing objects; alcohol odor; or other unusual behavior.

- *Interventions:* It is tough, but you have to stay calm; speak softly/slowly/clearly; respect patient's personal space; provide brief and honest facts; be an empathetic listener; encourage patient to verbalize feelings; provide "show of force" with security if needed; restrain as last resort; medicate as ordered and as necessary; and document all interventions and behaviors.
  - There are some people you cannot make happy no matter what you do. When you have tried everything listed previously, tell the person you will find someone to help and calmly *walk away!* Then chart the person's behavior and your interventions. Notify your charge nurse or supervisor that you require assistance.

Notes: _____

Psychosis

Psychosis is defined as a grossly impaired sense of reality. It is commonly associated with schizophrenia, which usually includes "negative symptoms," such as difficulty forming social and coherent conversations.

- *Causes:* Origin may be unknown, but the patient must be medically cleared. Some brain injuries, chemical imbalances, loss, separation, rejection, and use of illicit drugs can also cause psychosis.
- *Signs and symptoms:* Delusions; hallucinations; disorganized speech or behavior; catatonia; paranoia; poverty of speech; and flat affect.
- *Interventions:* Reorient to reality; maintain calm professional manner; explain unseen noises/voices/activities clearly and simply; give haloperidol (Haldol) as ordered; and respect patient's personal space.

Notes: _____

Fast Facts in a Nutshell

- Do not touch a patient who is hallucinating.
- The drug of choice for acute psychotic behavior is haloperidol (Haldol), administered by injection or intravenously.
- Large doses of haloperidol (Haldol) may prolong the Q-T interval; cardiac monitoring may be required.

Manic Behavior

Manic behavior is an elevated, unstable, or irritable mood. Bipolar disorder includes manic and depressive behaviors.

- *Causes:* Bipolar disorder and drug use are common.
- *Signs and symptoms:* Euphoria; grandiosity; insomnia; flight of ideas; aggression; easily distracted; impulsive; increased motor activity; and pressured speech (i.e., very talkative). You cannot get one word in with these patients.
- *Interventions:* Reduce stimuli; obtain urine drug screen and lithium level as ordered; reorient to reality; use "show of force" as needed with security personnel for aggressive behavior; set limits on manipulative/negative behavior; and restrain as needed for safety according to policy.

Notes: _____

Fast Facts in a Nutshell

A manic patient is at risk for harming himself or herself or others because of reckless behavior.

SUMMARY

You should now have a better understanding of mental health emergencies and how to handle them. From sad and suicidal patients to loud and schizophrenic patients wearing lampshades on their heads, you never know what kind of mental health challenge you will face next in the ED. Nevertheless, your mental health patients will respond better when you remain calm, speak concisely, respect personal space, and inform patients of upcoming procedures. *There are important legal issues and patient rights regarding mental health emergencies.* Document carefully and become familiar with your state's and facility's legal forms and policies regarding suicide, restraints, and seclusion. In addition, know how to get a hold of security personnel if you need them right away. You may find that mental health emergencies can be tough, sad, and rewarding.

15

Neurological Emergencies

The neurological system is a critical piece of the human puzzle. It is fascinating and fragile. There are many different forms of neurological emergencies. In the emergency department (ED), **you may see anything from head trauma with grand mal seizures to Bell's palsy.** It is important to get a good history and neurological assessment on these patients. This chapter helps you learn the major neurological emergencies and how to handle them.

During this part of your orientation, locate and become familiar with:

- Acute stroke protocol for your facility
- How to become National Institutes of Health Stroke Scale (NIHSS) certified online
- Neurological assessment tools (NIHSS and Glasgow Coma Scale)
- Tissue plasminogen activator (tPA) or (alteplase) administration guidelines
- Medications to know: Heparin, warfarin (Coumadin), nitroglycerin, sodium nitroprusside (Nipride), phenytoin (Dilantin), diazepam (Valium), and lorazepam (Ativan)

PLAN FOR THE WORST, HOPE FOR THE BEST

I will never forget a patient who took me by surprise. He came in unconscious and postictal from a witnessed seizure with no history available and no family. We were treating him for a routine seizure when he suddenly became hypertensive with multiple seizures, and we learned of his history of uncontrolled hypertension. He was having a massive hemorrhagic stroke—and not just a routine seizure! He needed a head CT scan super-stat!

DIAGNOSES

Acute Stroke (Cerebrovascular Accident)

A stroke is an interruption of cerebral circulation, also known as a "cerebrovascular accident." An acute stroke is marked by an onset of neurological symptoms within the past 48 hours and is considered a time-sensitive emergency. Time = brain tissue. The three classifications of strokes are listed in the following, along with their causes, manifestations, and interventions.

Ischemic

- *Causes:* Clot; thrombus; embolus; compression; or spasm. Large artery atherosclerosis, chronic hypertension, high cholesterol, obesity, atrial fibrillation, and diabetes contribute to ischemic strokes.
- *Signs and symptoms:* Usually occur while sleeping. Symptoms, which vary depending on location, magnitude, and duration, include arm drift; pupil changes; paralysis; facial droop; weakness; nausea and vomiting; hearing loss; headache; altered mental status; aphasia; dysphasia; receptive aphasia; visual disturbances; vertigo; ataxia; symptoms of increased intracranial pressure; and seizure.
- *Interventions:* Follow hospital stroke protocol (usually 3–4.5-hour window from onset of symptoms to treatment); maintain patent airway; monitor cardiac rhythm and blood pressure (BP); insert two large-bore intravenous (IV) accesses; administer oxygen; activate stroke team; obtain emergent CT scan of the head; give antihypertensive medications as ordered if systolic BP is greater than 185 mmHg and diastolic BP is greater than 110 mmHg (do not lower BP too fast!); perform coagulation studies, electrocardiogram, and frequent neurological assessments; and give anticoagulants (e.g., heparin, warfarin [Coumadin], antiplatelet medication [e.g., aspirin],

and thrombolytics [tPA, urokinase, and streptokinase]) as ordered.

Notes: _____

Hemorrhagic

- *Causes:* Rupture of cerebral blood vessel. Chronic hypertension, arteriovenous (AV) malformations, tumors, bleeding abnormalities, and aneurysm ruptures also contribute to hemorrhagic strokes.
- *Signs and symptoms:* Often occur suddenly upon waking or shortly thereafter. Symptoms, which vary depending on location, magnitude, and duration, include arm drift; pupil changes; paralysis; facial droop; weakness; nausea and vomiting; hearing loss; headache; altered mental status; aphasia; dysphasia; receptive aphasia; visual disturbances; vertigo; ataxia; symptoms of increased intracranial pressure; and seizure.
- *Interventions:* Follow hospital stroke protocol (usually 3–4.5-hour window from onset of symptoms to treatment); maintain patent airway; monitor cardiac rhythm and BP; administer oxygen; anticipate orders for CT scan of the head; give antihypertensive medications if systolic BP is greater than 185 mmHg and diastolic BP is greater than 110 mmHg (do not lower BP too fast!); and perform coagulation studies, glucose, electrocardiogram, and frequent neurological assessments. Consider surgical intervention. Prepare for operating room admission with neurosurgeon or transfer as ordered.

Notes: _____

Transient Ischemic Attack

A mini-stroke, also known as a "transient ischemic attack," is a temporary interruption of cerebral blood flow that resolves on its own.

- *Causes:* Temporary interruption of blood supply from a clot, spasm, or cerebral bleeding.
- *Signs and symptoms:* Symptoms, which vary depending on location, magnitude, and duration, persist less than 24 hours without permanent neurological deficit. They include arm drift; pupil changes; paralysis; facial droop; weakness; nausea and

Alteplase (tPA) DOOR TO NEEDLE GOAL ≤ 60 MIN

≤ 10 min	Support ABCs, ED provider and neurological assessment, blood glucose, IV access, activate stroke team, order head CT, EKG, and obtain labs
≤ 25 min	Establish symptom onset time, NIH stroke or Canadian neurological assessment, and head CT complete
≤ 45 min	CT and lab results interpreted, assess tPA exclusion criteria
≤ 1 hr	Review risks and benefits of fibrinolytic therapy, alteplase (tPA) bolus, and infusion given to eligible patients

Figure 15.1 National Institute for Neurological Disorders and Stroke (NINDS) time goals.

ABCs, airway, breathing, and circulation; ED, emergency department; IV, intravenous; NIH, National Institutes of Health; tPA, tissue plasminogen activator.

vomiting; hearing loss; headache; altered mental status; aphasia; dysphasia; receptive aphasia; visual disturbances; vertigo; ataxia; symptoms of increased intracranial pressure; and seizure.

■ *Interventions:* Follow hospital stroke protocol (usually 3–4.5-hour window from onset of symptoms to treatment; see Figure 15.1); maintain patent airway; watch cardiac and BP monitor; administer oxygen; anticipate orders for CT scan of the head, antihypertensive medications if systolic BP is greater than 185 mmHg and diastolic BP is greater than 110 mmHg (do not lower BP too fast!), coagulation studies, electrocardiogram, and frequent neurological assessments, and prepare for admission.

Notes: _____

Question: What is tPA?
Answer: *Tissue plasminogen activator (i.e., alteplase).*

It is a protein that helps convert plasminogen to plasmin, a major enzyme responsible for clot breakdown. It is approved only for ischemic strokes. *An accurate weight must be obtained.*

Fast Facts in a Nutshell

TPA Administration Key Points

- Establish two large-bore IV accesses.
- Complete inclusion/exclusion criteria checklist (see Table 15.1).
- Collaborate with your hospital or ED pharmacist to calculate a correct IV bolus and drip dose.
- Give tPA as early as possible.
  - Better outcomes within 1.5 hours than between 1.5 and 4.5 hours.
- Document frequent vital signs and neurological assessment during and post tPA administration according to hospital protocol.

Table 15.1

TPA Inclusion/Exclusion Criteria[a]

○ YES	Diagnosed with ischemic stroke causing measurable and disabling neurological deficit
○ YES	Onset of symptoms ≤3–4.5 hours
○ YES	Age ≥18 years of age
○ NO	Head trauma/stroke in past 3 months
○ NO	Subarachnoid hemorrhage symptoms
○ NO	Intracranial hemorrhage history
○ NO	Intracranial neoplasm/AV malformation/aneurysm/multilobar infarction
○ NO	Recent intracranial/intraspinal surgery
○ NO	Elevated BP ≥185/110
○ NO	Active or acute internal bleeding
○ NO	Takes anticoagulants with INR >1.7 or PT <15
○ NO	Blood glucose <50

[a]Provider may consider other relative exclusion criteria not listed in table.

AV, arteriovenous, BP, blood pressure; INR, international normalized ratio; PT, prothrombin time.

Fast Facts in a Nutshell

To triage a stroke, quickly just remember "FAST" assessment (**F**ace, **A**rm, **S**peech, and **T**ime).

During triage of a stroke patient, it is vital to assess the last known well time. This will help you determine if the stroke is acute.

Question: What do you give for warfarin (Coumadin) overdose?
Answer: *Vitamin K.*

Question: What do you give for heparin overdose?
Answer: *Protamine sulfate.*

Question: Patient states, "It is the worst headache of my life," and he has: nausea and vomiting; photosensitivity; hypertension; bradycardia; and aphasia. What is the most likely diagnosis?
Answer: *Ruptured cerebral aneurysm.*

Question: What are the guidelines for administering nitroprusside for hypertension?
Answer: *Protect from light with provided covering. Initial dose: 0.3 to a max of 10 mcg/kg/min.*

Seizures

A seizure is a sudden interruption of electrical brain activity, followed by a postictal state. Many different types are listed here, but the treatment is always the same.

- *Causes:* Aside from febrile seizures, the cause is not always known. Underlying conditions include brain tumor; cerebral infarct; head trauma; medication overdose; and alcohol abuse.
- *Signs and symptoms:* Each type of seizure, with specific signs and symptoms, is listed as follows:
  - *Generalized absence seizure (petit mal):* Characterized by staring or eyelid fluttering for 5 to 10 seconds.
  - *Tonic clonic (grand mal):* Generalized stiffening of extremities, followed by jerking movements; sweating; frothing at the mouth; incontinence; and amnesia.

- *Partial (focal):* Affects only part of the brain. Symptoms vary according to location of the seizure. It is usually accompanied by an aura. Focal seizures may be the result of underlying problems (e.g., trauma, tumor, or infarct).
- *Focal motor:* Starts with focal jerking that may persist or may spread to the entire body (grand mal).
- *Febrile:* Common in infants and young children with high fever.
- *Status epilepticus:* The seizure that never ends and is therefore an emergency! The patient keeps having one seizure after another so it looks like one long seizure. The patient with status epilepticus may have increased temperature, BP, and pulse. The patient is at risk for hypoxic brain damage.
- *Pseudoseizures:* When the patient is faking a seizure. Yes, this does actually happen! Patient movements may be purposeful, but the patient is not postictal after a fake seizure. This type of seizure is usually preceded by emotional upset, generally lasts longer than a true seizure, and the patient shows stable vital signs.
    - Arm Test: Hold the patient's arm above his or her face, and let go. A truly unconscious patient will hit his or her face with the arm. The pseudoseizure patient will avoid hitting the face.
    - Wave ammonia in front of the patient. If it is a pseudoseizure, the patient will suddenly be alert and oriented to person, place, and time.
- **Interventions:** Protect the patient from harm but do not restrain; protect airway; place in recovery position afterward; administer oxygen; anticipate orders to obtain an IV access, give medications (lorazepam, diazepam, and anticonvulsants), and reorient to reality after postictal state.

Notes: _____

Question: How fast do you give IV phenytoin (Dilantin)?
Answer: *Not faster than 50 mg/min using an in-line filter to avoid cardiac dysrhythmias and cardiac arrest. In addition, phenytoin (Dilantin) commonly causes phlebitis. If it infiltrates, it causes tissue necrosis!*

Question: Does phenytoin (Dilantin) treat petit mal seizures?
Answer: *No.*

(*continued*)

Question: What IV solution can be mixed with phenytoin (Dilantin)?
Answer: *Saline only (think seizure, think saline). Any other solution causes drug to crystallize.*

Question: Do febrile seizures cause permanent brain damage?
Answer: *No.*

Question: What can be mixed with diazepam (Valium) administered intravenously?
Answer: *Absolutely nothing, not even saline, as it will turn chalky.*

Bell's Palsy

Bell's palsy is paralysis of cranial nerve VII (facial). It usually resolves in several weeks to months.

- *Causes:* Unknown, but it is thought to be caused by a virus or immunodeficiency disorder.
- *Signs and symptoms:* Facial paralysis; headache; facial swelling; numbness; inability to close one eye; facial droop; and drooling.
- *Interventions:* Give medications (steroids, analgesics, artificial tears) as ordered and reassure the patient that he or she is not having a stroke.

Notes: _____

Myasthenia Gravis

Myasthenia gravis is a neuromuscular disorder.

- *Causes:* Thought to be caused by a myoneural junction defect.
- *Signs and symptoms:* Voluntary muscle weakness, especially of the face. Symptoms may improve with rest. Tensilon test is used to diagnose myasthenia gravis, as shown by the significant improvement of the patient after edrophonium is given intravenously.
- *Interventions:* Perform neurological assessments and give anticholinesterase drugs as ordered.

Notes: _____

Question: What is the antidote for anticholinesterase toxicity?
Answer: *Atropine.*

Multiple Sclerosis

Multiple sclerosis is a chronic autoimmune disorder in which the body attacks its own myelin sheaths, thereby damaging nerve impulses. The damage affects muscle coordination, strength, sensation, and vision.

- *Causes:* Unknown.
- *Signs and symptoms:* Diplopia; scotomas; tremor; blindness; weakness; fatigue; bladder/bowel incontinence; emotional instability; and paralysis.
- *Interventions:* Anticipate orders to administer diazepam, baclofen, and gabapentin to decrease spasms and tremors.

Notes: _____

Cluster Headache

A cluster headache is not one headache, but cycles of very painful headaches over 2 to 12 weeks.

- *Causes:* Unknown, but may be attributed to trigeminal nerve dysfunction.
- *Signs and symptoms:* Vary with the individual, but usually include intense pain on one side of the face or eye; runny nose; and nausea and vomiting. Usually, the patient has one tearing, puffy, red eye.
- *Interventions:* Give pain medication and administer 100% oxygen via nonrebreather for 7 to 8 minutes and then rest.

Notes: _____

Table 15.2

Glasgow Coma Scale

Eye opening	Verbal response	Motor response
4 spontaneously	5 orientated	6 obeys commands
3 to speech	4 confused	5 localized to pain
2 to pain	3 inappropriate	4 withdraws to pain
1 none	2 incomprehensible	3 flexion to pain
	1 none	2 extension to pain
		1 none

Fast Facts in a Nutshell

- The Glasgow Coma Scale (Table 15.2) assesses impaired consciousness by evaluating a patient's eye movement, body movement, and verbal responses. A patient with no eye movement, body movement, or verbal response would score a 3.
- Contraindications for lumbar puncture include taking warfarin (Coumadin); increased intracranial pressure; intracranial bleed; or infection of the lumbar puncture site.

SUMMARY

You now have a basic knowledge of neurological emergencies. You should be able to differentiate the various types and know how to treat them. Documenting a patient's complete history and neurological assessments is absolutely vital. Be familiar with your facility's neurological assessment tools, such as the NIHSS and Glasgow Coma Scale. Never underestimate your patient's symptoms. Sometimes a simple headache is the result of cerebral aneurysms, toxins, or brain masses. Therefore, concise assessments and rapid testing are key.

16

OB/GYN Emergencies

Obstetrical (OB) and gynecological (GYN) emergencies occur regularly in the emergency department (ED). As a nurse, you must be familiar and comfortable with the various types of OB/GYN emergencies. This chapter guides you through the many common types of OB/GYN challenges, including sexual assault, that you will face in the ED. When caring for these patients, be sure to always respect your patient's privacy by closing doors and curtains and providing blankets for covering up. Patients may be uncomfortable talking about OB/GYN matters. It is also true that some women are not well educated about their bodies. Some actually do deliver full-term babies in the ED without knowing they were pregnant. **Thus, the nurse must be sure to document a full and accurate triage, primary, and secondary assessment to find the source of the patient's complaint.** You may have to ask a lot of questions to get the necessary patient history. Always be prepared for the possibility and challenges of caring for two patients in one package: mother and baby or babies.

During this part of your orientation, locate and become familiar with:

- Precipitous delivery tray
- Pelvic examination equipment and specimen supplies
- Doppler for fetal heart tones
- Facility's policy and procedure for sexual assault, OB in the ED, methotrexate administration, and RhoGAM administration

(continued)

- Evidence collection kit
- Medications to know: Ceftriaxone (Rocephin), azithromycin (Zithromax), RhoGAM injection, and methotrexate

DIAGNOSES

Endometriosis

Endometriosis is a painful menstrual cycle that occurs because endometrial tissue fragments are found outside the uterus.

- *Causes:* The abnormal tissue fragments react to hormones and slough during menstruation, thereby causing pelvic pain.
- *Signs and symptoms:* Pelvic pain with menstruation; dysuria; irregular menstrual cycles; and abnormal uterine bleeding.
- *Interventions:* As ordered, administer analgesic medication and evaluate effectiveness; bed rest; set up and assist in pelvic examination; refer patient to OB/GYN specialist.

Notes: _____

Bartholin's Cyst

Bartholin's cyst is an obstruction/abscess of the Bartholin gland. The Bartholin gland is responsible for vaginal secretions during sexual arousal.

- *Causes:* Sexually transmitted infection or swelling can cause a clogged or obstructed Bartholin gland.
- *Signs and symptoms:* Pain with intercourse and vaginal lump or abscess.
- *Interventions:* Anticipate orders to administer analgesic/narcotic medications and document effectiveness, prepare for incision and drainage, assist with Word catheter insertion, administer antibiotics, and teach patient about sitz baths.

Notes: _____

Table 16.1

Causes of Vaginitis	
Bacterial vaginosis	**Candida albicans**
Gray–white, thin, fish-odor vaginal discharge	White, curd cheese–like vaginal discharge
Give metronidazole or clindamycin by mouth	Give medications fluconazole (Diflucan) by mouth or miconazole intravaginal

Vaginitis

"Vaginitis" is a general term for an altered vaginal flora pH.

- *Causes:* Acquired immunodeficiency syndrome; allergic reaction; bacterial vaginosis; *Trichomonas vaginitis*; foreign object (e.g., old tampon); and yeast (*Candida albicans*) infection.
- *Signs and symptoms:* Red inflamed vaginal mucosa and abnormal vaginal discharge (see Table 16.1).
- *Interventions:* Prepare for pelvic exam with culture specimen collection as ordered; administer medication according to offending organism; pelvic rest; and patient teaching.

Notes: _____

Pelvic Inflammatory Disease

Pelvic inflammatory disease (PID) is a vaginal bacterial infection that ascends into and beyond the cervix.

- *Causes:* Usually starts as a vaginal bacterial infection that spreads into and beyond the cervix.
- *Signs and symptoms:* Fever; lower abdominal pain with rebound tenderness; irregular menstrual cycle; foul-odor vaginal discharge; cervical inflammation; "the PID shuffle," shuffling gait due to pain; elevated white blood cell count; and severe pain on pelvic examination.
- *Interventions:* Prepare cultures for pelvic exam; bed rest; anticipate orders to administer analgesic/narcotic pain medications, evaluate pain medication and document effectiveness, give

fluids intravenously or by mouth, administer antibiotics, and teach patient about pelvic rest and prevention.

Notes: _____

Question: Which microorganism is the most common cause of PID? **Answer:** *Neisseria gonorrhea.*

Long-term complications related to under- or untreated PID may include increased risk for ectopic pregnancy and infertility. Discharge instructions should include an emphasis on completion of therapy and follow-up care with gynecologist.

Sexual Assault

"Sexual assault" is an assault of a sexual nature to another person, or any sexual act committed against someone's will. It comes in many forms. Most frequently, sexual assaults are committed by a man against a woman. Although less frequent, sexual assault can and does occur to men and children as well.

Rape is the coerced or forced penetration of the vulva or anus with a penis, an object, or any other body part.

It is highly recommended that you take a sexual assault class or become a sexual assault nurse examiner (SANE) to fully understand how to care for the sexually assaulted patient.

- *Causes:* Not all causes are known. However, research shows that sexual assault is sometimes used as an expression of dominance and/or power over the person being assaulted. High-risk behavior of the male perpetrator includes use of drugs or alcohol, lack of inhibitions, history of sexual abuse, sexual promiscuity, associating with sexually aggressive friends, limited economic resources, hostility toward women, and lack of emotional support.
- *Signs and symptoms:* Vary based on the type of sexual assault. Obtaining a good history is critical, as not all sexual assaults will leave visible injuries. Your patient may or may not be tearful and anxious. You may or may not note bruising, lacerations, abrasions, or patterned marks on the patient. Reports of memory loss are not uncommon, and may indicate the victim is suffering from a toxicological emergency as well. Be aware of this

possibility and implications of drug and alcohol screening in criminal proceedings.

- *Interventions:*
    - Review your facility's policy and procedure for sexual assault.
    - During triage, assess and document the patient's safety and injury, and obtain an accurate, nonjudgmental history in a private location. Use of quotations for subjective data can be helpful. The patient should not wait in the waiting room; triage the sexual assault patient as a higher priority according to your hospital policy.
    - Explain assessments, treatment plans, and options with the patient.
    - Determine whether the patient wants to file a police report and whether he or she wants evidence to be collected.
    - Before you ask the patient to change into a patient gown, remember the clothing the patient is wearing might be evidence. If the clothing was worn during the sexual assault, place two flat sheets on the floor and ask the patient to stand in the middle of the sheet and completely undress. Don gloves to put the underwear in a small paper bag labeled "underwear." Ask the patient to step off the sheet. Then place each item of clothing in separate, small, labeled paper bags. Next place all bagged and labeled clothing and the top sheet in a large paper bag. Seal, staple, and label the large paper bag with the patient's name.
    - Provide privacy and comfort measures such as a blanket, hospital socks, tissues; allow a friend to stay with patient; and allow normal elimination.
    - Perform a complete head-to-toe assessment documenting the injury type, patterned marks, size, shape, number, and location, and whether any penetrating or blunt force trauma occurred. Do not assume anything. Leave your opinions out; document only what you see. Know that your documentation may be used in court.
    - If the patient wants evidence to be collected, obtain an evidence collection kit. Be sure to collect everything you need before you open the kit (e.g., pelvic exam equipment, sterile scissors, and sterile water). Once the kit is open and collection begins, you must maintain the chain of custody. Chain of custody guidelines require that samples and kits are correctly secured and documented before they can leave your presence. Follow instructions on the kit or according to your facility's policy and procedure. Collections may vary based on

type of assault. In general, the order of collection looks something like this:

- ❑ Head hair samples
- ❑ Oral swabs
- ❑ Fingernail cuttings and scrapings
- ❑ Other secretions, stains, or forensic material
- ❑ Pubic hair samples
- ❑ Vaginal/cervical samples (collected by a provider or SANE team member via pelvic exam)
- ❑ Anal or rectal samples

Notes: _____

Fast Facts in a Nutshell

Myth: There will always be visible injuries when someone is "really" sexually assaulted.
Reality: Not all sexual encounters cause visible injuries.
Myth: Rape is usually committed by a stranger.
Reality: Most rape victims are raped by a family member or an acquaintance in a private location.

Ectopic Pregnancy

An ectopic pregnancy occurs when a fertilized egg implants anywhere outside of the uterus (usually in the fallopian tubes). Complications include a ruptured ectopic pregnancy and hemorrhage.

- *Causes:* The cause is not always known, but PID with scarring and tubal ligation are contributing factors.
- *Signs and symptoms:* Unilateral severe sharp pelvic pain is a high alert for impending/imminent rupture. Cramping or minimal pain may occur in the earlier stages. Absent or slight vaginal bleeding; irregular or missed period; positive pregnancy test; positive Kehr's sign; and signs of shock if fallopian tube is ruptured.
- *Interventions:* Anticipate orders to perform pregnancy test, check human chorionic gonadotropin (Hcg) level, arrange for pelvic/transvaginal ultrasound, start large-bore intravenous access, set up pelvic examination, perform coagulation studies, type and screen blood, determine Rh factor, check frequent vital signs, and prepare for methotrexate administration or surgery.

- *Complication:* Rupture of the fallopian tube may cause bleeding into the pelvic cavity. Occult bleeding may not be obvious; pain is a hallmark sign. This is a surgical emergency, and significant, uncontrolled bleeding may lead to hypovolemic shock.

Notes: _____

Spontaneous Abortion (Miscarriage)

Miscarriage occurs before the age of viability (20th week of gestation). Table 16.2 shows the various types of miscarriages: complete, incomplete, threatened, inevitable, septic, and missed. Complications include infection and hemorrhage.

Notes: _____

Question: A 22-year-old female arrives in the ED complaining of right lower quadrant abdominal pain. What must be ruled out?
Answer: *Ectopic pregnancy, kidney stones, and appendicitis.*

Note: One saturated pad or tampon = 5 to 15 mL of blood.

RhoGAM may be ordered for Rh-negative women demonstrating signs and symptoms of ectopic pregnancy and/or spontaneous miscarriage. This product helps desensitize the mother's body, when there is possibility of fetal Rh-positive blood mixing with maternal Rh-negative blood. Such mixing of positive and negative blood could cause a hemolytic reaction, similar to mismatched blood transfusions. RhoGAM may be dispensed from pharmacy or lab, depending on your facility's policy. It is important to know the policies, process, and guidelines for administration and documentation at your hospital.

Placenta Previa

Placenta previa occurs when the placenta implants itself in the lower uterus, thereby partially or completely covering the cervical opening.

- *Causes:* Unknown.
- *Signs and symptoms:* Painless bright-red vaginal bleeding during pregnancy, and soft nontender abdomen.

Table 16.2

Types of Miscarriages

	Threatened	Complete	Incomplete or inevitable	Septic	Missed
Symptoms	Slight vaginal bleeding Mild uterine cramps Closed/slightly opened cervix Intrauterine pregnancy on US Fetal heart tones	Slight vaginal bleeding No uterine cramps Closed cervix No intrauterine pregnancy on US All products of conception have passed	Severe vaginal bleeding and clots Moderate uterine cramps Open cervix Ruptured amniotic membranes	Foul vaginal dc/bleeding Severe abd/pelvic pain Fever; chills Open cervix	Slight vaginal bleeding Closed cervix No fetal heart beat or intrauterine products of conception noted on US
Interventions	Pelvic exam Pelvic US RhoGAM injection if Rh is negative Bed and pelvic rest[a] OB/GYN follow-up CBC	Pelvic exam Pelvic US RhoGAM injection if Rh is negative Bed and pelvic rest[a] CBC OB/GYN doctor follow-up	Pelvic exam Pelvic US RhoGAM injection if Rh is negative Bed rest CBC Type and screen Pelvic rest[a] OB/GYN follow-up	Pelvic exam/US Blood cultures; CBC IV antibiotics Recheck vital signs RhoGAM injection if Rh is negative Bed and pelvic rest[a] IV fluids and oxytocin Possible D&C OB/GYN follow-up	Pelvic exam Pelvic US Coagulation studies Bed and pelvic rest[a] OB/GYN follow-up Possible surgical intervention

[a]Pelvic rest means no sexual intercourse, no tampons, and nothing inside vagina.

abd, abdominal; CBC, complete blood count; D&C, dilation and curettage; dc, discharge; IV, intravenous; OB/GYN, obstetrical and gynecological; US, ultrasound.

- *Interventions:* Anticipate orders to provide bed rest, start large-bore intravenous access, monitor fetal heart tones and frequent vital signs, count menstrual pads, monitor for signs of shock, position the patient on left lateral side, arrange for pelvic ultrasound, type and crossmatch, and complete blood count. ***Pelvic exam is contraindicated, as it could cause further bleeding.*** **Get the patient to the birth center** and prepare for possible emergency C-section. Remember, "If the bleeding is bright and new, you **cannot** do," the pelvic exam.

Notes: _____

Abruptio Placentae

Abruptio placentae occurs when the placenta breaks away from the uterine wall before delivery.

- *Causes:* Not always known, but can be attributed to abdominal trauma or a very short umbilical cord pulling on the placenta.
- *Signs and symptoms:* Abdominal pain/cramps; profuse or concealed *dark-red vaginal bleeding;* backaches; uterine contractions; fetal distress; and signs of shock.
- *Interventions:* Position patient on her left side; administer high-flow oxygen via nonrebreather mask; monitor fetal heart tones, frequent vital signs, and cardiac rhythm; anticipate orders to: begin large-bore intravenous access; perform coagulation studies; complete blood count; type and screen blood; prepare for possible emergency C-section and blood transfusion; and notify and transport to birth center or the operating room.

Notes: _____

Question: What is the major difference between placenta previa and abruptio placentae?
Answer: *Placenta previa has painless bright-red vaginal bleeding; abruptio placentae has painful dark-red vaginal bleeding.*

PREGNANCY-INDUCED HYPERTENSION OR GESTATIONAL HYPERTENSION

Pregnancy-induced hypertension is diagnosed hypertension that occurs only during pregnancy, usually after the 20th week. Once the pregnancy is over, the blood pressure is normotensive again. Systemic vasoconstriction may compromise both the placenta and fetal circulation.

Preeclampsia

Preeclampsia is a pregnancy complication characterized by gestational hypertension plus proteinuria.

- *Causes:* Unknown.
- *Signs and symptoms:* Hypertension; headaches; edema; epigastric pain; sudden weight gain; proteinuria; double vision; uterine contractions; and vaginal bleeding.
- *Interventions:* Monitor blood pressure; perform urinalysis; arrange for transvaginal or pelvic ultrasound; order bed rest; position patient on left side; monitor urine output; anticipate orders to obtain a complete metabolic panel, a complete blood count, and a liver function test; monitor cardiac performance and fetal heart tones; begin intravenous access; prepare for possible hospital admission; take seizure precautions; obtain OB consultation; and consider administering intravenous magnesium sulfate.

Notes: _____

Eclampsia

Eclampsia is a seizure associated with preeclampsia. This is an emergency! During a seizure, circulation of oxygen and nutrients may be compromised to mother and fetus.

- *Causes:* Unknown.
- *Signs and symptoms:* Seizure activity associated with preeclampsia symptoms, including hypertension; headaches; edema; epigastric pain; sudden weight gain; proteinuria; double vision; uterine contractions; and vaginal bleeding.
- *Interventions:* Anticipate orders to begin intravenous access; take serum uric acid and liver function tests; perform a complete blood

count and basic metabolic panel; measure hourly urine output via Foley catheter; administer anticonvulsants intravenously (e.g., magnesium sulfate); administer hydralazine intramuscularly or intravenously if diastolic blood pressure is greater than 110 mmHg; monitor cardiac performance, level of consciousness, urinary output, and blood pressure; take seizure precautions; provide psychosocial support; consult with OB; notify labor and delivery units; and prepare for emergent delivery.

Notes: _____

Prolapsed Cord

The cord is prolapsed when a pregnant woman comes into the ED in active labor and you see the cord hanging out. **Get her to the birth center immediately.**

- *Causes:* Unknown.
- *Signs and symptoms:* A woman in active labor with the umbilical cord presenting through the vaginal canal before the baby.
- *Interventions:* Do *not* try to put the cord back in. Manual pressure can be applied to the baby's head by gently pushing up with the finger to relieve pressure on umbilical cord. Manual pressure may need to be maintained until appropriately relieved. Prepare for emergency C-section. Maternal positioning with hips up and head down may help relieve fetal pressure on the cord, but monitor and ensure maternal airway, breathing, and circulation are not compromised.

Notes: _____

Trauma During Pregnancy

This trauma is the result of an injury that occurred during pregnancy.

- *Causes:* Vary individually. Shift in weight and unsteady gait contribute to falls and injuries during pregnancy. Be alert for the possibility of interpersonal violence.
- *Signs and symptoms:* Vary depending on the injury. May include vaginal bleeding, ruptured membranes, or even abdominal asymmetry if uterine rupture.
- *Interventions:* Assess uterine contractions and fetal heart tones (normal is 120–160 beats/min); place the patient in left lateral

recumbent position; anticipate orders to obtain large-bore intravenous access; administer isotonic intravenous fluids; determine presence of any amniotic fluids with pH strip; inspect vaginal opening for crowning; check for any fetal movement; palpate and determine fundal height; arrange for pelvic or transvaginal ultrasound and CT scan; perform coagulation studies; prepare a complete blood count; type and screen blood; arrange for pelvic examination; assess breath sounds for pulmonary edema; prepare for blood transfusion; and prepare for emergency C-section. *No* vasopressors due to fetal compromise.

Notes: _____

Fast Facts in a Nutshell

- If a pregnant patient is on a backboard, tilt the client to her left side to move the uterus off the inferior vena cava.
- Consider early blood transfusion. Large quantities of isotonic fluids do not improve fetal hypoxia.
- A pregnant trauma patient can lose up to 30% of blood volume before becoming hypotensive.

Emergency Delivery

It is rare, but sometimes babies are delivered in the ED. Most times, we feel ill prepared. Sometimes patients do not know they are pregnant or are in denial. Just remember, women have been delivering babies naturally without hospitals and nurses since the beginning of time.

- *Causes:* There are only three reasons to deliver a baby in the ED. (1) The patient in active labor did not know she was pregnant. (2) The patient is miscarrying and is less than 20 weeks pregnant. (3) The active labor patient accidentally comes to the ED instead of to the birthing center and delivers prior to being transferred to the birthing center.
- *Signs and symptoms:* "Bloody show" or loss of mucus plug; amniotic fluid leakage; crowning or a visible baby's head; and an uncontrollable desire to push (patient may ask to use the bathroom).
- *Interventions:* Position the patient on her left side; administer oxygen; and visually check for crowning. If signs of imminent

delivery are present, be prepared to "catch" the baby; obtain intravenous access as ordered; monitor fetal heart tones and contractions; and prepare for **rapid vaginal examination unless vaginal bleeding is present**. Vaginal bleeding due to placenta previa may cause **life-threatening hemorrhage.**

- *Infant resuscitation:* You have caught the baby; now what? Call for help if you do not have any. You now have two patients, so you need one nurse for the mother and one for the infant.
- *Prevent heat loss by drying the baby* and wrapping him or her in warm blankets/towels; use warming light; and place baby directly against mother's chest and cover both.
- *Suctioning:* Bulb suction mouth, then nose. If you do not have bulb suction, use wall suction with oral Yankauer adapter.
- *Provide oxygen:* If neonatal oxygen levels do not steadily rise above 94% within 10 minutes of delivery (see Table 16.3).
- *Stimulate:* If the drying and the suction do not work, rub the infant's back or flick/slap soles of feet. If still not breathing, use bag valve mask to assist ventilations.
- *The Apgar score* is used to determine fetal status. Use Table 16.4 to determine the baby's score. You want the baby to score a perfect 10.

Notes: _____

Question: Where would a 32-week-pregnant patient diagnosed with appendicitis be hurting?
Answer: *Right upper quadrant because the appendix gets pushed up later in pregnancy.*

Question: What does "gravida" mean? What does "para" mean?
Answer: *"Gravida" means the number of pregnancies. "Para" means the number of live births.*

The Neonatal Resuscitation Program (NRP) may also benefit the ED nurse on the assessment, interventions, and specific care needs of infants intra- and postdelivery, and during the neonatal stage of life (0–30 days).

Table 16.3

Target Neonatal Room Air Oxygen Levels Postdelivery	
1 minute	60%–65%
2 minutes	65%–70%
3 minutes	70%–75%
4 minutes	75%–80%
5 minutes	80%–85%
10 minutes	85%–95%

Table 16.4

The Apgar Score			
Sign	0	1	2
Color	Cyanotic/blue	Body pink, blue extremities	Whole body pink
Muscle tone	Limp	Some flexion	Active movement
Respirations	Absent	Slow, irregular	Good (30–60 bpm)
Heart rate	Absent	Slow (less than 100 bpm)	Good (100–180 bpm)
Reflex irritability (tactile stimulation)	No response	Facial grimace	Cry, cough, sneeze

SUMMARY

You should now have a more detailed knowledge base of obstetrical and gynecological emergencies. Be sure to locate and be familiar with all your obstetrical and gynecological equipment. Nothing is worse than running around trying to find supplies during an emergency. Be sure to practice assisting with a couple of pelvic examinations during your orientation. At first, you may feel like you need a few extra hands to assist with the examinations. Obtain a good history! This means asking questions, such as when did it start, does anything make the pain worse, how many pads did you go through today? With pregnant patients, consider the fact that you may have two or more patients. Always be professional and respect your patient's privacy.

17

Ocular Emergencies

You will come across a variety of eye emergencies working in the emergency department (ED). Some are as simple as pink eye, whereas others require emergency ophthalmic surgery. **As a nurse, you must be able to differentiate between nonurgent and emergent eye complaints.** This chapter guides you through the various types of eye emergencies and teaches you the manifestations and interventions for each. Be sure to practice with the eye supplies available at your facility during your orientation. Familiarization with your supplies will enable you to obtain a thorough eye assessment of your patients. The providers with whom you work will be expecting a visual acuity test on all eye complaints. **Document carefully and keep your eyes open**—you never know what you will see next in the ED.

During this part of your orientation, locate and become familiar with:

- Wood's lamp, slit lamp, Tono-Pen or tonometer
- Eye exam supplies (fluorescein strips, tetracaine or proparacaine hydrochloride [Alcaine] eyedrops)
- Visual acuity charts
- pH indicator strips
- Morgan lens and eye irrigation supplies
- Gentamicin ophthalmic ointment
- Eye patches

- All patients with eye complaints need to have their visual acuity documented.
- OS is left eye. OD is right eye. OU is both eyes.

DIAGNOSES

Central Retinal Artery Occlusion

This is a thrombus or embolus central retinal artery occlusion. There is a *1-hour* window to restore blood flow. **This is a true ocular emergency!**

- *Causes:* Just as with a stroke, thrombi or emboli can occlude the retinal artery, cutting off the blood supply to the eye.
- *Signs and symptoms:* Sudden/painless/unilateral/complete loss of vision; dilated nonreactive pupil; and pale fundus.
- *Interventions:* Check the patient's visual acuity; obtain eye exam equipment; anticipate orders to obtain intravenous access, administer vasodilators (e.g., intravenous nitroglycerin) and anticoagulants, arrange ophthalmology consult, and prepare for surgery.

Notes: _____

Glaucoma

Acute open-angle glaucoma occurs from optic nerve damage.

- *Causes:* It starts with blockage of the outflow of fluid from the anterior chamber. This results in elevated intraocular pressure leading to optic nerve damage.
- *Signs and symptoms:* Diminished vision; deep eye pain; nausea and vomiting; tearing; photophobia; cloudy cornea; semidilated nonreactive pupils; red conjunctiva; and increased ocular pressure.
- *Interventions:* Perform visual acuity test; anticipate provider will monitor ocular pressure; administer myotic eyedrops/topical beta antagonists as ordered; and obtain ophthalmologist consult.

Notes: _____

Corneal Abrasions

These are scratches/abrasions to the clear surface (cornea) of the eye with or without foreign bodies.

- *Causes:* Practically anything that can scratch the skin can scratch the cornea. In most cases, abrasion is caused by some type of foreign body.
- *Signs and symptoms:* Eye pain; corneal irregularity; no corneal luster; photophobia; copious tearing; and foreign body sensation.
- *Interventions:* Assess visual acuity; obtain eye exam equipment (eye kit, Wood's lamp); anticipate orders to administer antibiotic eyedrops or ointment, update tetanus/diphtheria shot, administer oral analgesics, and provide ophthalmologist referral.

Notes: _____

Detached Retina

The retina is made of two layers (outer pigmented and inner sensory). A detached retina occurs when these layers separate.

- *Causes:* Vitreous humor leakage; eye trauma; inflammatory disorders; and uncontrolled diabetes.
- *Signs and symptoms:* Painless decreased vision; smoky or cloudy vision; flashing lights; and peripheral floaters (black dots)/"curtain effect."
- *Interventions:* Check visual acuity; position patient supinely; anticipate orders to arrange ophthalmology consult, administer mydriatic drops to dilate pupil, apply bilateral eye patches, and prepare for surgery and admission.

Notes: _____

Conjunctivitis/Pink Eye

This is an inflammation of the conjunctiva. Bacterial and viral conjunctivitis are highly contagious.

- *Causes:* Bacteria, viruses, chemicals, or allergies.
- *Signs and symptoms:* Itchy eyes; photophobia; normal visual acuity; purulent or serous eye discharge; reddened conjunctiva; and copious tearing.

- *Interventions:* Assess visual acuity; anticipate orders to instill topical anesthetic, obtain fluorescein staining supplies and Wood's lamp, and instill ophthalmic antibiotic eyedrops or ointment.

Notes: _____

Fast Facts in a Nutshell

Because conjunctivitis is so contagious, discharge instructions should include strict hand washing after touching eye area, no sharing of hand towels, discarding current eye makeup, and disinfecting sunglasses.

Penetrating Trauma

Penetrating trauma requires immediate ophthalmology consult. Protruding objects are *not* to be removed, but carefully secured in place.

- *Causes:* These vary. You name it, but anything from knives and bullets to nails shot through nail guns have been seen in the ED. Practically anything with enough force behind it can cause penetrating trauma to the eye.
- *Signs and symptoms:* Irregular pupil shape; impaired visual acuity; and decreased intraocular pressure.
- *Interventions:* Prepare for ophthalmology consult; cover injured eye with metal or plastic patch and patch other eye to reduce eye movement; put patient in semi-Fowler's position; anticipate orders to administer pain medication and give tetanus/diphtheria injection.

Notes: _____

Blunt Trauma Blow-Out Fractures

This is a fracture of the orbital floor.

- *Causes:* Inferior orbital rim trauma.
- *Signs and symptoms:* Change in gaze; diplopia; ecchymosis; subconjunctival hemorrhage; paresthesia; periorbital edema; crepitus; and inability to look up due to inferior rectus/inferior oblique muscle entrapment.

- *Interventions:* Apply ice pack; anticipate orders to administer pain medications, arrange for orbital x-rays or CT scan, put patient in semi-Fowler's position, and prepare for possible admission or surgery.

Notes: _____

Hyphema

Hyphema is a hemorrhage into the anterior chamber of the eye that results in corneal blood staining, secondary glaucoma, visual impairment, or loss of an eye.

- *Causes:* Eye trauma.
- *Signs and symptoms:* Blood in anterior chamber of eye; impaired visual acuity; and "seeing red" or floater.
- *Interventions:* Elevate the patient's head of the bed to 60°; gently patch both eyes; anticipate orders to arrange immediate ophthalmology consult, monitor intraocular pressure, and administer mannitol or osmotic diuretic for increased intraocular pressure.

Notes: _____

Chemical Burns

Chemical burns are the result of contact with *acid* or *alkali* solutions. Alkali is more serious and can result in loss of vision. **This is a true eye emergency!**

- *Causes:* Foreign chemical contact with the eye.
- *Signs and symptoms:* Eye pain; visual disturbances; corneal whitening; copious tearing; surrounding skin irritation; and corneal ulceration.
- *Interventions:* Assess visual acuity; check pH with litmus paper; immediately apply copious amounts of normal saline/lactated Ringer's; anticipate orders to maintain continuous irrigation until pH of the eye is 6.9 to 7.2, administer ophthalmic ointment, and arrange ophthalmology referral.

Notes: _____

Acid burns usually require 30- to 60-minute irrigations. Alkali burns may take 1 hour or longer to irrigate. This procedure gets fluid everywhere. You will need to give the patient a gown and a towel and have him or her lie on the stretcher; place the patient in slight Trendelenburg position. Then place a basin on the floor at the head of the bed. Finally, place a couple of Chux folded like a funnel that drain into a basin on the floor.

SUMMARY

Eye emergencies occur pretty routinely in the ED. It is vital to recognize which ones are emergent and which ones are nonurgent. Be sure to document pupil size, pupil reaction to light, pupil symmetry, and visual acuity. You should now be more confident in recognizing the symptoms and treatments for the various types of eye emergencies and in treating them. However, you need to practice with the current eye supplies at your facility to truly complete your ocular emergency orientation.

18

Orthopedic and Wound Care Emergencies

You will definitely see all kinds of orthopedic and wound emergencies in the emergency department (ED). You need to be familiar with many different pieces of orthopedic equipment. In addition to using the equipment, the ED nurse is also responsible for teaching the patient how to use the orthopedic equipment. For casts of Ortho-Glass type splinting, I recommend training from the manufacturer's representative. **Most manufacturers will send someone to your facility to demonstrate their products and allow employees to practice applying the splints.** Most ED technicians are qualified to apply splints for you, but the nurse must ensure the work was done properly. Assess and document circulation, motion, and sensation before and after splinting. This chapter provides a brief overview of the different orthopedic and wound care emergency situations you may come across in the ED, and how to handle them.

During this part of your orientation, locate and become familiar with:

- Ace wraps, splinting, and casting materials
- Crutches
- Hare traction splints and Buck's traction
- Tube gauze and hemostatic gauze
- Finger traps and weights

(continued)

- Suture supplies and dressing supplies
- Medications to know: Lidocaine 1% or 2% (with or without epinephrine), bupivacaine (Marcaine) with or without epinephrine, morphine, hydrocodone (Lortab), oxycodone (Percocet), and acetaminophen (Tylenol) with codeine

DIAGNOSES

Strains

A strain is a pull or tear to a tendon or muscle.

- *Causes:* Injury resulting in a pull or tear to a tendon.
- *Signs and symptoms:* Pain; swelling; ecchymosis; edema; point tenderness; spasm; and decreased range of motion.
- *Interventions:* Mnemonic: **PRICE** (**P**rotect [splint, cast, sling], **R**est, **I**ce, **C**ompression [ace wrap], **E**levate); x-ray; instruct patient on use of crutches for light to no weight bearing; and arrange orthopedic follow-up.

Notes: _____

Sprains

A sprain is a pull or tear to a ligament, commonly in the knees, ankles, and shoulders.

- *Causes:* Injury resulting in a pull or tear to a ligament.
- *Signs and symptoms:* Pain; swelling; ecchymosis; edema; point tenderness; spasm; and decreased range of motion.
- *Interventions:* Mnemonic: PRICE; x-ray; instruct patient on light to no weight bearing (crutches); and arrange orthopedic follow-up.

Notes: _____

Fractures

A fracture is a broken bone or disruption in normal continuity of bone, cartilage, or both.

Chapter 18 Orthopedic and Wound Care Emergencies

- *Types:*
  - Closed: Skin intact.
  - Open: Broken bone with break in the skin surrounding the fracture. Patient is at high risk for developing an infection in the bone (osteomyelitis).
  - Avulsion: Insertion site bone fragment breaks away due to forceful muscle contraction.
  - Comminuted: Two or more bone fragments.
  - Depressed: Flat bone injury due to blunt trauma.
  - Greenstick: Incomplete compression force-type fracture (common in school-age children).
  - Spiral: Twisting injury.
  - Oblique: Linear oblique fracture.
  - Transverse: Horizontal linear fracture.
  - Segmented: Broken in two or more places.
  - Salter–Harris: Fracture involving the growth plate.
  - Boxer fracture: Occurs to the fourth or fifth metacarpals after punching type injury.
- *Causes:* Injury or disease process resulting in a break to the bone. Consider corresponding injuries to surrounding tissue, nerves, blood vessels, or internal organs.
- *Signs and symptoms:* Pain; tenderness; swelling; redness; ecchymosis; deformity; shortening/rotation in hip fracture; decreased range of motion; muscle spasm; weak or absent pulses; pallor; and shock.
- *Interventions:* Administer pain medication promptly as ordered and document effectiveness; immobilize; assist in applying traction for femur fracture; remove any rings or jewelry to the fractured extremity; cover open fractures with sterile saline-soaked dressing; mnemonic: PRICE; x-ray; no weight bearing (crutches); prepare for possible closed reduction; give nothing by mouth; give instructions for possible surgical repair; teach cast care instructions and crutch training; check peripheral pulses; anticipate orders to start intravenous access; possibly give intravenous fluids and tetanus immunization if open fracture; and arrange orthopedic follow-up.

Notes: _____

Question: Pneumothorax or great vessel injury may occur with which type to fracture?
Answer: *Clavicle (collar bone) fracture.*

Question: How long does it take a bone to heal?
Answer: *About 6 weeks.*

Question: What other x-ray should be ordered for the patient who has bilateral heel fractures after falling 13 feet off a ladder and landing on his feet?
Answer: *Check the L-spine.*

Question: Which bones, if broken, can lead to hemorrhagic shock?
Answer: *Pelvis and femur.*

Question: How much blood can be lost in one femur fracture?
Answer: *Up to 1,500 mL.*

Question: When applying a thumb spica Ortho-Glass splint, how should you position the hand?
Answer: *As if the patient were holding a cup or soda can.*

Dislocations and Subluxations

Dislocations and subluxations occur when a joint is pulled out of place.

- *Causes:* Injury or movement resulting in joint dislocation.
- *Signs and symptoms:* Severe joint pain; joint deformity/asymmetry; decreased or absent range of motion; weak or absent pulse; edema; and shortening of extremity.
- *Interventions:* Anticipate orders to obtain x-ray films, prepare for conscious sedation for closed reduction, apply ice pack, start intravenous access, prepare a neurovascular assessment, immobilize joint postreduction, and obtain postreduction x-ray.

Notes: _____

Amputation

Amputation is a partial or complete separation of a limb.

- *Causes:* Injury/trauma resulting in separation of a limb.
- *Signs and symptoms:* Completely or partially detached extremity.

- *Interventions:* Treat airway, breathing, and circulation (ABCs) first. Administer oxygen and initiate two large-bore intravenous accesses. Wrap amputated part in sterile saline-soaked gauze and place in sterile plastic bag or container. Place bag or container on crushed ice and water. **Never put amputated part directly on ice.** Control bleeding; apply sterile saline-soaked sterile dressing to amputation site; anticipate orders to administer pain meds/ antibiotics/tetanus immunization and evaluate effectiveness of medications; and prepare for surgery.

Notes: _____

Fast Facts in a Nutshell

Do not forget to properly label the amputated part.

Compartment Syndrome

This occurs when a compartment of the limb becomes full of fluid or blood, thereby hindering circulation to that extremity.

- *Causes:* Usually occurs with trauma.
- *Signs and symptoms:* The five **P**s: **P**ain, **P**aresthesia, **P**ulseless, **P**aralysis, and **P**allor.
- *Interventions:* Administer anti-inflammatory drugs as ordered; elevate the affected limb; and prepare for emergency fasciotomy. Discharge teaching should include instructions to return for any increasing pain, pallor, or decreased circulation below the cast or splint.

Notes: _____

Lacerations Versus Cuts

Lacerations are breaks or tears in the skin due to blunt trauma. Cuts occur from sharp objects.

- *Causes:* Everything from pieces of glass, knives, and razors to umbrellas, coffee tables, and baseball bats. You name it; almost anything can cause a laceration or cut.

- *Signs and symptoms:* Bleeding, cut, and open wound. An arterial laceration will intermittently squirt blood with each pulse. If a vein is cut, it will constantly ooze. Superficial lacerations are easily repaired in the ED. Deep wounds through the muscle fascia or tendons may require a plastic surgeon.
- *Interventions:* Apply pressure to control bleeding; update tetanus shot if greater than 5 years since last one; cleanse wound with chlorohexidine soap; prepare patient for wound closure with Dermabond, Steri-strips, or sutures per provider order; bandage accordingly.

Notes: _____

Question: When setting up for suture repair of the ear, nose, penis, fingers, or toes, should you use lidocaine with epinephrine?
Answer: *No.*

Question: What supplies are needed for suture set-up?
Answer: *Suture tray, sutures, povidone-iodine (Betadine)/ChloraPrep, saline, lidocaine, Chux, and sterile gloves.*

Question: What are two shots that can be given in the deltoid?
Answer: *Tetanus/diphtheria and the flu shot.*

Burns

A burn is a breakdown in the skin.

- *Causes:* Chemicals; sun; heat; radiation; fire; or even cold substances such as dry ice.
- *Signs and symptoms:*
  - *First degree:* Superficial pink color or redness; pain; and warmth to area.
  - *Second degree:* Redness; blistering; break in first layer of skin down to second layer of skin; and pain.
  - *Third degree:* White areas or charred black areas to skin; painless; all layers of skin affected; and possibly fat, muscle, and bone involvement.
- *Interventions:* Check ABCs first. Patient may have smoke/burn inhalation or carbon monoxide poisoning. Cover minor burns

with sterile nonadhesive dressings; give pain medication as ordered; cleanse burns with chlorohexidine soap and saline; and apply silver sulfadiazine (Silvadene) cream, and nonadherent dressings. Screen the patient for possible abuse. If it is a major burn, prepare for admission to burn center.

Notes: _____

Question: Why are wet-to-dry dressings contraindicated in patients with major burns?
Answer: *Wet-to-dry dressings may cause hypothermia.*

Figure 18.1 shows the "rule of nines" for adult burn victims. This is a fast way to determine a patient's percentage of burned surfaces using multiples of nine.

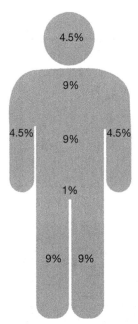

Figure 18.1 Rule of nines.

SUMMARY

You now have a better understanding of orthopedic and wound care emergencies, their symptoms, and treatments. Be sure to familiarize yourself with the orthopedic and wound care supplies at your local facility. Thoroughly document your assessments, being sure to include distal pulses, capillary refills, deformities, symmetry, whether bleeding is controlled, and when and how the injury occurred. Use personal protective equipment, especially with arterial bleeds. Arterial bleeds have been known to squirt across the room. In case this happens and your clothes get soiled, it is also a good idea to keep an extra pair of scrubs in your locker. Teach patients the importance of an orthopedic follow-up; the ED visit goal is to stabilize, and small fractures may not be visible until swelling subsides.

19

Pediatric Emergencies

Children can be some of the most delightful and yet scariest patients you will ever meet. Why scary? For two reasons. First, **children cannot always tell you what is wrong.** So you must assess them well and listen to parents. Although sometimes challenging, **family-centered care is crucial,** and parents generally know when something is wrong with their babies. Second, **children may look okay when they are actually in distress** because they are good at compensating. When they can no longer compensate, they deteriorate rapidly. This is called the "plateau effect." This does not leave the emergency department (ED) staff with much time to resuscitate them. Therefore, you must treat children aggressively at the early signs of distress, which include tachycardia and increased respirations. Hypotension is a late sign, which is followed by rapid deterioration. You will learn about this extensively during your pediatric advanced life support course. **Pediatric emergency nursing really is a specialty of its own,** but this chapter provides you with some of the basic pediatric emergency nursing tools you will need.

During this part of your orientation, locate and become familiar with:

- Broselow tape and cart/bag
- Where to take a pediatric advanced life support class or emergency nurse pediatric course (ENPC)
- Kilogram/pound conversion

(continued)

- Pediatric acetaminophen (Tylenol) and ibuprofen (Motrin) doses
- Pediatric vital signs
- Papoose board
- Intraosseous needle, also known as "IO needle," placement and use
- Review Emergency Medical Treatment and Labor Act (EMTALA) and hospital policy for consent to treat minors
- Stickers, popsicles, crayons, flashlights, and toys, as these are great for passing time and bribing

Fast Facts in a Nutshell

When children deteriorate, they generally deteriorate more rapidly than adults.

- Pediatric emergencies account for about 20% to 30% of all ED visits in United States.
- The majority are seen in nonpediatric EDs.
- Injuries are fifth leading cause of death in children younger than 1 year of age, after perinatal conditions, congenital abnormalities, sudden infant death syndrome (SIDS), and heart conditions.

Table 19.1 lists all of the pediatric vital signs according to age group. You will need to know these by heart, so it is a good idea to familiarize yourself with these vital signs during your orientation. Basically, the younger the child, the lower the blood pressure and higher the heart rate and respirations will be.

Fast Facts in a Nutshell

Obtain blood pressure in children 4 years of age and older. Do not use the words "blood pressure," as it scares them. Tell them you are going to give their arm a hug with an arm-hugging machine or check their arm muscles.

Table 19.1

Age-Specific Normal Vital Signs

Age	Newborn	Infant	Toddler	Preschooler	School age	Adolescent	Adult
Respirations	40–60	30–63	22–37	20–28	18–25	12–20	12–20
Heart rate	90–205	90–180	80–140	65–120	58–115	50–100	60–100
Systolic blood pressure	67–84	72–104	86–106	89–112	97–115	110–131	120

FEVER

In children, a fever is defined as a rectal temperature of 100.4°F or higher. Infants younger than 3 months of age with fever are at high risk for having a serious bacterial infection, such as sepsis or meningitis. A febrile child without an obvious source of fever requires an extensive evaluation and possible admission.

- *Causes:* Otitis media; pneumonia; viral/bacterial infections; gastroenteritis; bacteremia; meningitis; and upper respiratory infections.
- *Signs and symptoms:* Poor feeding; rectal temperature greater than 100.4°F; irritability; lethargy; dry mucous membranes; decreased tear production; sunken or bulging fontanel; tachycardia; and tachypnea.
- *Interventions:* Anticipate orders to give antipyretic medications (acetaminophen [Tylenol] = 15 mg/kg, ibuprofen [Motrin] = 10 mg/kg) by mouth or suppository, administer intravenous fluids for dehydration, and monitor temperature.

Notes: _____

Fast Facts in a Nutshell

- Sepsis work-up in infants younger than 3 months of age includes labs, chest x-ray, and lumbar puncture. Remember when positioning patient for a lumbar puncture, there should be no chin to chest, as this might occlude the airway. Instead, curve shoulders (not the head) forward.
- Fluids after a lumbar puncture may prevent headache in a young child.
- Children's ibuprofen (Motrin) is not given to children younger than 6 months of age.
- A 4-year-old with gastroenteritis who is discharged from the emergency department should be encouraged to drink small sips of clear liquids as much as he or she can tolerate to make up fluid loss. Popsicles and Jell-O are kid-friendly choices.

EPIGLOTTITIS

Epiglottitis is a rapid swelling and inflammation of the epiglottis that can lead to a life-threatening airway obstruction. It commonly occurs in children 2 to 6 years of age.

- *Causes:* Acute bacterial infection of the epiglottis.
- *Signs and symptoms:* Sudden onset (2–4 hours); drooling; dysphagia or refusing to drink; inspiratory stridor (abnormal sound over trachea); respiratory distress; tripod position; muffled voice; hoarseness; high fever; sore throat; and anxiety.
- *Interventions:* Decrease stimulation (do not make them cry); maintain position of comfort; permit caregiver to stay with child; give oxygen by any method tolerated (blow-by); anticipate orders to prepare for intubation or emergency tracheostomy, start intravenous access after securing airway, and administer antibiotics.

Notes: _____

BRONCHIOLITIS

Bronchiolitis is a viral infection of the bronchioles, with increased mucous secretion that results in mucus plugging and air trapping.

- *Causes:* The respiratory syncytial virus. It mostly affects infants younger than 1 year of age.
- *Signs and symptoms:* Cough; runny nose; poor feeding; respiratory distress; pallor; retractions; grunting; nasal flaring; wheezing; apnea spells; and fever.
- *Interventions:* Anticipate orders to: arrange for chest x-ray; administer fluids by mouth or intravenously; isolate; give oxygen; use nebulizers; administer racemic epinephrine, ribavirin; place head of bed up; and prepare for admission, if severe.

Notes: _____

CROUP

Croup is inflammation and edema of the vocal cords, trachea, and bronchi. It most commonly affects children from 6 months to 3 years of age at night in late fall to early winter.

- *Causes:* A viral illness.
- *Signs and symptoms:* Barking cough (*like a barking seal*); inspiratory stridor; hoarse voice; respiratory distress; low fever; and tachycardia.
- *Interventions:* Anticipate orders to administer cool-mist oxygen, give fluids by mouth or intravenously, and give steroids and racemic epinephrine.

Notes: _____

Fast Facts in a Nutshell

Pediatric intramuscular (IM) injection tips

- Do *not* use deltoid.
- Best site is anterolateral thigh.
- Get everything ready (adhesive bandages, alcohol swabs); bring a colleague to help hold the child.
- Due to volume, most antibiotic IM injections must be divided into two shots and given simultaneously.

SHUNTED HYDROCEPHALUS

Hydrocephalus is commonly caused by obstructed cerebrospinal fluid, which leads to a dilated ventricular system. A shunt is inserted to drain the fluid away from the cranium to the peritoneum or the left atria. Ventriculoperitoneal shunts are the most common. A child might present to the ED as a result of infection or malfunction of the shunt.

- *Causes:* Obstruction to flow of cerebrospinal fluid.
- *Signs and symptoms:* Fever; behavioral changes; erythema or fluid along shunt tubing track; meningeal signs; acute abdominal pain; diarrhea; peritonitis; increased intracranial pressure; seizure activity; and headache.

- *Interventions:* Maintain support of airway, breathing, and circulation (ABCs); elevate head of bed up 30°; anticipate orders to administer intravenous fluids (often fluid is restricted), diuretics, analgesics, anticonvulsants, and antibiotics and monitor their effectiveness; anticipate need of removal of cerebrospinal fluid from shunt; take seizure precautions; and monitor cardiac performance, respiratory rate, and continuous pulse oximetry.

Notes: _____

CHILD MALTREATMENT

Remember that child maltreatment includes physical, emotional, psychological, and sexual abuse, as well as neglect.

- *Causes:* Many nurses find it impossible to understand what causes a person to harm a child, but it can happen in any socioeconomic class and is usually brought on by the adult's inability to cope with stress.
- *Signs and symptoms:* Bruises or fractures in various stages of healing; burn patterns from cigarettes or hot water; human bite marks; head injuries from direct blows or vigorous shaking, alopecia, lip bruising or laceration; loss of teeth; hyphema; corneal abrasion; retinal hemorrhage; orbital fracture; periorbital hematoma; spiral fractures from twisting injuries; and abdominal trauma (abdominal distention, nausea and vomiting, and abdominal pain).
  - A history may provide vital clues. Always interview parents individually, and, if possible, the child separately.
    - Is there any preexisting medical condition that explains present injuries?
    - Does caregiver's history match the mechanism of injury?
    - Does caregiver deny knowledge of injury occurrence?
    - Are there any inconsistent history changes?
    - Was there any delay in seeking medical attention?
    - Is there any history of unexplained suspicious injuries?
    - Has the caregiver bypassed closer medical facilities to reach yours?
    - Is anyone else besides the parents caring for the child?
- *Signs and symptoms of neglect:* Malnourishment; poor hygiene; inappropriate dress; inadequate medical care; bald patches on

infant head from being left in crib in one position for long time; abandonment; numerous dental problems; lack of supervision; and educational neglect.

- *Signs and symptoms of sexual abuse:* Genital/rectal trauma; vaginal/rectal bleeding or pain; vaginal discharge; unusual vaginal/rectal dilation; increased rectal pigmentation; dysuria; frequent urination; foreign bodies in vagina/urethra/rectum; pregnancy; difficulty ambulating; sexually transmitted diseases; and bowel incontinence.

- *Interventions:* Anticipate orders to perform labs (HIV, rapid plasma reagin, amylase, and lipase); arrange for CT scan, ultrasound, and x-rays (complete skeletal survey in child younger than 2 years of age); provide safe environment; treat injuries; provide emotional support to caregiver and child; remain nonjudgmental; explain tests and procedures; allow caregiver to remain with child except during interview; refer to social services; report all suspected cases to child protective services; complete appropriate paperwork; carefully document shape, size, location, and appearance of all injuries; and document reports from caregiver and child word for word in quotation marks. For suspected sexual abuse, lab protocol may include collecting vaginal/cervical/rectal culture; vaginal/rectal fluids; pregnancy test; ABO-antigen typing; and hair specimen.

Notes: _____

Fast Facts in a Nutshell

- Parents from any socioeconomic class may be child abusers.
- The abused child does not cry when parent leaves the room.

Question: Which is not considered child abuse?
   a. Burns from the ankles down
   b. Missing hair on head
   c. Belt marks
   d. Bruises on bilateral elbows and knees
Answer: *d is correct.*

CONGENITAL HEART DISEASES

There are several different types; they are classified as left-to-right shunts (acyanotic) or right-to-left shunts (cyanotic).

- Left-to-right shunts (acyanotic): Atrial septal defect, atrioventricular septal defect, ventricular septal defect, and patent ductus arteriosus.
- Right-to-left shunts (cyanotic): Tetralogy of Fallot, tricuspid atresia, transposition of the great vessels, aortic stenosis, pulmonic stenosis, and coarctation of the aorta.
  - *Causes:* Unknown.
  - *Signs and symptoms:* Cyanosis with feeding or activity; decreased urine; edema; cardiomegaly; hepatomegaly; developmental delays; murmurs; tachycardia; bradycardia; tachypnea; dyspnea; cough; respiratory distress; clubbing of fingers or toes; poor peripheral circulation; mottling of extremities; syncope; and "tet spells" (squatting position to relieve dyspnea).
  - *Interventions:* Remember the ABCs; provide basic life support if indicated; anticipate orders for arterial blood gas levels, electrocardiogram and echocardiogram, possible cardiac catheter procedure; allow child to be in position of comfort; administer oxygen; use bag valve mask if needed; start intravenous access; set head of bed at 30°; administer medications (digitalis, diuretics, analgesics, and sedatives) as ordered; limit noxious stimuli; and keep comfortably warm.

Notes: _____

NURSEMAID'S ELBOW (RADIAL HEAD SUBLUXATION)

Nursemaid's elbow is a subluxation of the elbow.

- *Causes:* Commonly occurs when a child younger than 5 years of age is grabbed by the forearm to pull up or swing.
- *Signs and symptoms:* No use of suspected arm after pulling mechanism of the forearm. Child may guard arm. No signs of trauma noted.
- *Intervention:* Assist with simple reduction, arrange for x-ray, administer analgesics as ordered, and apply ice pack.

Notes: _____

SUDDEN INFANT DEATH SYNDROME

This is the most common cause of death in infants between 1 month and 1 year of age.

- *Causes:* Unknown. Studies show that placing an infant on his or her back to sleep helps reduce the risk of sudden infant death syndrome.
- *Signs and symptoms:* Most caregivers report finding an infant in a crib not breathing or face down in crib. Autopsy fails to reveal cause of death.
- *Interventions:* Attempt to resuscitate using pediatric advanced life support protocol, unless obvious rigor mortis has set in. *Refer parents to sudden infant death syndrome support group.*

Notes: _____

INTUSSUSCEPTION

Intussusception occurs when a segment of the intestines folds over on itself like a telescope. It most commonly occurs in children younger than 1 year of age. Intussusception can lead to obstruction, edema, and bowel necrosis.

- *Causes:* Unknown; although existing medical conditions may be factors.
- *Signs and symptoms:* Change in eating or bowel pattern; colic; crying; drawing up knees; vomiting; currant-jelly–like red stool; recent infection; and palpable sausage-like mass.
- *Interventions:* Anticipate orders to use nasogastric tube for decompression, administer intravenous fluids, give antibiotics, and prepare for surgical reduction if needed.

Notes: _____

Fast Facts in a Nutshell

- After visiting her grandfather who has shingles, a little girl develops a rash. The rash is most likely chickenpox.

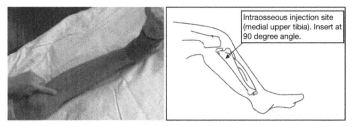

Figure 19.1 Proximal medial tibia: Primary pediatric intraosseous site location.

Figure 19.1 is a picture of an IO injection site. This site is primarily used if intravenous access is unobtainable after attempting for 30 seconds during an emergency situation.

SUMMARY

Pediatric emergency nursing is its own specialty. For the general emergency nurse, the basic information in this chapter will see you through most problems. Be sure to always take account of differences between children and adults. Pediatric patients have different vital signs, deteriorate more rapidly than adults, become dehydrated more easily, and can run higher fevers. All pediatric patient medication doses are based on weight in kilograms. Remember that children cannot always tell you what is wrong. Therefore, it is up to the nurse to obtain an accurate history and detailed physical assessment. If you are ever unsure of something, ask a coworker or go find the answer. The pediatric patient is not just a patient; he or she is someone's child! Sometimes the toughest challenge is defusing the hysterical parent's anger or anxiety. Parents do not always realize they are hindering or delaying care when they panic. If the situation cannot be defused, do not waste time. Have another coworker or manager handle the parent, leaving you to care for the child. You now have the knowledge base to diagnose and handle pediatric emergencies. Be careful: These little patients know how to pull on your heart strings.

20

Respiratory Emergencies

Of all emergencies, respiratory problems must be treated first. **Without a patent airway and breathing, your patient will die—and nothing else matters.** Therefore, as an emergency nurse, you must be able to recognize and rapidly respond to any respiratory emergency. This chapter takes you through the most common respiratory conditions seen in the emergency department (ED). After reviewing it, you will be able to recognize the various types of respiratory emergencies and know how to intervene.

During this part of your orientation, locate and become familiar with:

- Ambu-bags, nasal cannulas, nonrebreather masks, and nebulizers
- Intubation or cricothyrotomy equipment
- Chest tubes and drainage systems
- Ventilators, bilevel positive airway pressure (BiPAP), and continuous positive airway pressure (C-PAP)
- Reading arterial blood gases
- Medications to know: Methylprednisolone sodium succinate (Solu-Medrol), dexamethasone (Decadron), levofloxacin (Levaquin), magnesium sulfate, albuterol, ipratropium bromide (Atrovent), and levobuterol hydrochloride (Xopenex)

Fast Facts in a Nutshell

Always treat airway first, breathing next, and then circulation. Just remember ABC.

It is important to recognize when a patient is in respiratory distress or respiratory failure; however, these terms are often misused.

- Respiratory distress: results in *decreased* oxygenation and/or ventilation
- Respiratory failure: results in *inadequate* oxygenation and/or ventilation

DIAGNOSES

Acute Respiratory Distress Syndrome (ARDS)

ARDS affects children and adults. It is brought about by alveolar histamine release after lung injury resulting in a fluid shift into alveoli and inhibiting surfactant. The result is poor gas exchange, atelectasis, pulmonary edema, hypoxemia, and possible alveolar collapse or fibrosis.

- *Causes:* Near drowning, aspiration, trauma, infection or sepsis, toxins, heroin, cocaine, acute pancreatitis, metabolic disturbances, burns, fat embolism, disseminated intravascular coagulation (DIC), and hematologic disorders.
- *Signs and symptoms:* Severe rapid onset of dyspnea; restlessness; crackles; rhonchi; tachycardia; low pulse oximetry reading despite oxygen therapy; hypoxia; tachypnea; and pulmonary infiltrates on chest x-ray.
- *Interventions:* Anticipate orders to assist ventilations, rapid sequence intubation (RSI); monitor pulse oximetry/wave form capnography; provide high-flow oxygen; obtain intravenous access; obtain portable chest x-ray, arterial blood gas (ABGs), and serum lactate levels.

Notes: _____

Fast Facts in a Nutshell

To remember ARDS, use the following mnemonic:

Assault to lung tissue
Released histamine
Damaged alveoli
Severe respiratory failure

Airway Obstructions

These can be divided into partial, complete, and upper or lower airway obstructions.

- *Causes:* Vary depending on circumstance. Anything from food to coins to a swollen tongue can occlude an airway.
- *Signs and symptoms:* Respiratory distress; dyspnea; choking sensation; drooling; wheezing; decreased or no air movement; aphasia; tachycardia; tachypnea; cough; chest retractions; pallor or cyanosis; and cardiopulmonary arrest.
- *Interventions:* Clear airway; initiate basic life support techniques for foreign-object obstruction; anticipate foreign body removal with Magill forceps by provider and orders to administer oxygen; measure pulse oximetry; if alert and coughing, place in high Fowler's position of comfort; prepare for intubation and possible cricothyrotomy or tracheostomy; document airway patency changes; and document respirations frequently.

Notes: _____

Question: A child swallowed a quarter, is drooling, and has an unusual cough. What is your concern?
Answer: *Airway obstruction (remember your ABCs).*

When medicating for RSI, always administer sedatives prior to paralytics.

Assisting With RSI

RSI is a technique used to paralyze and sedate an alert or semiconscious patient just prior to performing endotracheal intubation. This process is usually performed by a team including an ED provider, respiratory therapist, and an advanced cardiovascular life support (ACLS) certified registered ED nurse.

RSI Preparation Checklist

- Attach cardiac, pulse oximeter, blood pressure, and continuous wave form capnography device to patient.
- Establish intravenous or intraosseous access.
- Provide oxygen supply to patient via nonrebreather mask. Have bag valve mask ready.
- Suction equipment is available and working properly.
- Nasal or oral pharyngeal airways are available in appropriate sizes.
- Endotracheal tubes with stylets are available in appropriate sizes.
- Laryngoscope with curved or straight blades are available and working (and video laryngoscope).
- 10-mL syringe to test inflate endotracheal balloon is available.
- Endotracheal securement device or cloth tape is available.
- Crash cart is in room.
- Rescue or difficult airway equipment is available.

RSI Step by Step

- Prepare equipment (see checklist previously).
- Open airway (maintaining C-spine immobilization if injury present).
- Pre-oxygenate patient with 100% oxygen via nonrebreather or bag valve mask.
- Anticipate orders to premedicate as indicated for increased risk of bradycardia or increased intracranial pressure:
  - Atropine (Atropen): Adults: rescue dose; pediatrics: 0.01 to 0.02 mg/kg (max 0.5) to inhibit bradycardia response.
  - Fentanyl: Adults: 1 to 3 mcg/kg; pediatrics: 1 mcg/kg to prevent intracranial pressure increase during RSI.
  - Lidocaine (Xylocaine): Adults: 100 mg (2% 5-mL syringe); pediatrics: 1.5 mg/kg (max 100 mg) to prevent intracranial pressure, and suppress cough reflex during RSI.
- Anticipate orders to administer sedation or anesthesia IV push. Examples are as follows:
  - Etomidate: 0.3 mg/kg
  - Fentanyl citrate (Sublimaze): 2 to 10 mcg/kg

- Ketamine (Ketalar): 1 to 2 mg/kg
- Midazolam (Versed): 0.1 to 0.3 mg/kg (max 10 mg)
- Propofol (Dipravan): 1 to 2 mg/kg. Check state law for RN administration conditions
- Thiopental (Thiopental): 2 to 5 mg/kg
- Anticipate orders to administer paralytic or neuromuscular blocking agent IV push. Ensure provider is fully prepared to intubate prior to pushing any of these drugs, as the patient will *stop* breathing once it is given! Examples are as follows:
  - Succinylcholine (Anectine): 1 to 1.5 mg/kg. Increases potassium and causes bradycardia. Contraindicated in renal, hyperkalemic, bradycardic, burn, or crush injury patients.
  - Vecuronium: 0.1 to 0.2 mg/kg
  - Rocuronium (Zemuron): 1 mg/kg
- Provider will assess whether patient is relaxed enough to intubate. Look for jaw relaxation and apnea.
- Monitor continuous pulse oximeter, wave form capnography, and vital signs while provider attempts endotracheal intubation.
- If intubation is successful, provider will inflate balloon. If provider is unsuccessful, be ready to assist ventilations with bag valve mask.
- Confirm placement by attaching bag valve mask to endotracheal tube to listen for bilateral breath sounds; listen to ensure there are no epigastric sounds; attach CO_2 detection device; and monitor wave form capnography.
- Secure endotracheal tube with cloth tape or commercial securement device.
- Document time, confirmed placement methods, endotracheal tube size, and tube placement at the lip. A respiratory therapist will usually attach ventilator to endotracheal tube at this time.
- *Continue sedation* and frequent vital sign monitoring.

Notes: _____

Chronic Obstructive Pulmonary Disease

Chronic obstructive pulmonary disease (COPD) is an irreversible chronic obstructive small airway disease. A patient with COPD will have elevated carbon dioxide levels. Over time, the elevated carbon dioxide levels will make the patient dependent on lower PAO_2 level changes (hypoxia) to regulate ventilations. Therefore, if you deliver high-flow oxygen for an extended period of time, the patient will lose his or her hypoxic respiratory drive *and stop breathing!*

- *Causes:* Enlargement of the alveoli, loss of lung tissue elasticity, and destruction of alveolar wall. This chronic lung damage is associated with emphysema, chronic bronchitis, and cigarette smoking.
- *Signs and symptoms:* Dyspnea; tachypnea; pursed-lip breathing; wheezing; crackles; tripod position; use of accessory muscles; barrel chest; tachycardia; hypertension; confusion; cyanosis; premature ventricular contractions; and acute respiratory failure.
- *Interventions:* Anticipate orders to: obtain and monitor arterial blood gases, administer 1 to 2 L of low-flow oxygen because of carbon dioxide retention, position head of bed up 90%, apply BiPAP, give nebulizer treatments and corticosteroids, and give high-flow oxygen via nonrebreather only if patient is in severe respiratory distress.

Notes: _____

Asthma

Asthma is a reversible chronic reactive airway disease. It is a complex inflammatory response characterized by large airway inflammation and structural changes. Asthma is classified into four categories. Decrease in oxygen level is a late sign.

- *Causes:* A hypersensitive immune system reaction that causes the airways to inflame and swell when exposed to certain triggers. The triggers vary from person to person, but common triggers include dust, pollen, pet dander, exercise, cigarette smoke, medications (aspirin or NSAIDs [nonsteroidal anti-inflammatory drugs]), upper respiratory infections, and gastroesophageal reflux disease.
- *Signs and symptoms:* Vary by category.
  - *Mild intermittent:* Expiratory wheezing; pulse oximeter reading of 95% to 100%; and cough.
  - *Mild persistent:* Inspiratory and expiratory wheezing; pulse oxygen of 95% to 100%; and cough.
  - *Moderate persistent:* Inspiratory wheezing; expirations diminished; cough; use of accessory muscles; retractions; nasal flaring; and tripod position.

- *Severe persistent:* Expirations and inspirations diminished (silent lung); no breath sounds; diaphoresis; dusky pallor or cyanotic skin color; pulse oxygen reading of less than 95%; bradypnea or periods of apnea; and drowsiness or altered mental status.
- *Interventions:* Position for comfort; anticipate orders to give oxygen, nebulizer treatment, steroids, and magnesium sulfate; hydrate the patient; apply BiPAP; and intubate in late stages.

Notes: _____

Fast Facts in a Nutshell

- As bronchospasms improve or reverse, breath sounds go from diminished to louder to clear.
- Diphenhydramine hydrochloide (Benadryl), propranolol (Inderal), or morphine sulfate may be contraindicated in asthmatic patients. Benadryl can dry and thicken mucus. Inderal can block bronchodilation. Morphine can cause respiratory depression.
- The optimal peak expiratory flow rate is greater than 80% of predicted or personal best.

Spontaneous Pneumothorax

Spontaneous pneumothorax is an air leak in the pleural space that results in partial or total collapse of the lung.

- *Causes:* Not always known. However, COPD, asthma, cystic fibrosis, tuberculosis, pneumonia, lung cancer, interstitial lung disease, inhaled substance abuse, barometric pressure changes (scuba divers, pilots), ingestion of toxic drug pentamidine, smoking, and immunodeficiency disease all attribute to spontaneous pneumothoraxes.
- *Signs and symptoms:* Dyspnea; tachypnea; tachycardia; sudden pleuritic chest pain; anxiety; restlessness; diminished or absent breath sounds on affected side; pallor; hypotension (if severe); subcutaneous emphysema; palpitations; or asymptomatic (if small).
- *Interventions:* Place in high Fowler's position; prepare for needle thoracostomy, Heimlich valve, or chest tube insertion; and administer pain meds as ordered.

Fast Facts in a Nutshell

If a tall, thin young adult states, "I suddenly coughed and became short of breath," think spontaneous pneumothorax.

Pneumonia

Pneumonia is an acute inflammatory reaction that results in fluid and cellular debris accumulating in segments and lobes of the lung.

- *Causes:* Aspiration, bacterial, mycoplasmas, fungi, foreign material, or viral infections.
- *Signs and symptoms:* Productive cough; green, bloody, or rust color sputum; fever (acute onset); chills; pleuritic chest pain; dyspnea; tachypnea; respiratory distress; tachycardia; confusion; altered level of consciousness; crackles; wheezing; diminished breath sounds; and weight loss.
- *Interventions:* Anticipate orders to obtain intravenous access, obtain blood cultures, administer antibiotics, rehydrate, use nebulizers, order complete blood count and chest x-ray, and give antipyretics (if fever).

Notes: _____

Question: What is the major pulmonary cause of septic shock?
Answer: *Acute bacterial pneumonia.*

Burn Inhalation

If a patient has burns to the face, consider the possibility of burns to the large and small airways. Patients may appear stable initially, but remember that burns swell quickly, resulting in rapid loss of airway.

- *Causes:* Burns to face, neck, chest, mouth, or airway.
- *Signs and symptoms:* Black-tinged sputum; dry mucous membranes; rales; rhonchi; and dry nonproductive cough. Singed nasal hair, eyebrows, and eye lashes.

- *Interventions:* Prepare for emergent intubation, apply nonre-breather oxygen mask, and anticipate order to obtain arterial blood gases.

Notes: _____

SUMMARY

You now have a strong foundation to assess and treat respiratory emergencies. Be sure to thoroughly document respiratory assessments. This should include rate, depth, breath sounds, symmetry, skin color, use of accessory muscles (if labored or unlabored), and ability to speak in full sentences before and after each intervention. It is imperative that you are competent in recognizing and treating all respiratory emergencies. To make you more comfortable with respiratory problems, be sure to familiarize yourself with all your facility's respiratory supplies and equipment. Knowing where your supplies are and how to use them will make your job easier. If you have a lot of questions, a respiratory therapist can be a good resource. Never forget: In any emergency, treat the airway first, then breathing, and then circulation.

21

Shock and Multisystem Trauma Emergencies

Patients in shock or with multisystem trauma are considered critical, so a knowledge of these emergencies is vital for the emergency department (ED) nurse. The window of opportunity to save these patients' lives is small. In this chapter, you will learn the various forms of shock and how to intervene. You will also gain a better understanding of multiple types of trauma and how to manage them. Be sure to learn your facility's trauma protocols and be familiar with any trauma or shock supplies. It is also highly recommended that you sign up for and take the Trauma Nurse Core Course. It is a valuable certification to have and will help increase your knowledge in this area.

During this part of your orientation, locate and become familiar with:

- Rapid infusers, blood warmers, blood tubing, and blood bank
- Protocols for sepsis, mass transfusions, and uncross-matched blood transfusions
- Trauma and therapeutic hypothermia policies and protocols
- C-spine immobilization devices
- Anaphylactic drug supply box
- Chest tubes, thoracentesis tray, chest tube drainage systems, Heimlich valve, and autotransfusers
- Tourniquet application

(continued)

- Medications to know: Dopamine, norepinephrine (Levophed), epinephrine, dobutamine, milrinone, phenylephrine, vasopressin methylprednisolone sodium succinate (Solu-Medrol), dexamethasone (Decadron), diphenhydramine hydrochloride (Benadryl), and famotidine (Pepcid)

DIAGNOSES

Shock

Remember that shock simply means "inadequate tissue perfusion," despite the cause.

There are three stages to any form of shock.

- *Compensated:* This is the early phase of shock in which the body compensates for the decreased tissue perfusion with vasoconstriction, tachycardia, decreased urine output, and tachypnea, as blood pressure remains normotensive. **Early recognition and interventions during this phase can improve mortality rates by about 70%.**
- *Uncompensated or hypovolemic:* This stage is marked by hypotension and signs of poor circulation. The body can no longer compensate to maintain adequate tissue perfusion and blood pressure.
- *Irreversible or refractory:* This stage is marked by symptoms of cellular, tissue, organ or multiorgan death and dysfunction. Poor patient outcomes and death are common despite aggressive treatments and interventions.

There are four types of shock:

- Hypovolemic (most common)
  - Hemorrhagic
  - Nonhemorrhagic (dehydration)
- Cardiogenic
- Obstructive
  - Cardiac tamponade
  - Tension pneumothorax
  - Massive pulmonary embolism

- Distributive
  - Septic
  - Anaphylactic
  - Neurogenic

Hypovolemic Shock

This is a decrease in circulating volume. Hypovolemic shock is the most common form of shock in a trauma patient. **Control any external hemorrhage;** hemorrhage is one of the most preventable causes of death.

- *Causes:* Lack blood volume because of laceration of a major blood vessel; gastrointestinal bleeding; severe dehydration; ruptured organ; severe burns; crush injuries; bleeding aneurysm; and poor clotting factors.
- *Signs and symptoms:* Hypotension; narrowing pulse pressure; tachycardia; and altered level of consciousness. Early signs and symptoms may include restlessness, anxiety, and confusion.
- *Interventions:* Assess and treat any external hemorrhage, then treat airway, breathing, and circulation (ABCs); monitor vital signs, cardiac performance, and oxygen levels; anticipate orders to obtain two large-bore intravenous (IV) accesses, administer warmed IV crystalloid fluid infusion of 20 to 40 mL/kg, prepare transfusion of whole or packed red blood cells and fresh frozen plasma or platelets, and apply direct pressure or tourniquet to profusely bleeding lacerations.

Notes: _____

Question: In a pediatric patient, what are some late signs of hypovolemic shock?
Answer: *Bradycardia, hypotension. Cyanosis and tachycardia are early signs.*

Question: A patient with hyperosmolar hyperglycemic nonketotic syndrome is at risk for what type of shock?
Answer: *Hypovolemic shock.*

Question: What is the only IV fluid that can be infused with blood?
Answer: *Normal saline.*

Cardiogenic Shock

In cardiogenic shock, the heart fails to pump blood effectively.

- *Causes:* Myocardial infarction; dysrhythmias; cardiac failure; blunt cardiac trauma; or myocardial contusion.
- *Signs and symptoms:* Hypoxia; anxiety; diaphoretic and rapid weak pulse; dysrhythmias; jugular vein distention (JVD); hypotension; S3 heart sound; pulmonary edema; crackles; and tachypnea.
- *Interventions:* Treat ABCs. Anticipate orders to apply cardiac monitor, open two large-bore IV accesses, administer oxygen, take electrocardiogram and pulse oxygen, administer IV fluid bolus cautiously and administer appropriate antiarrhythmic medications, treat the underlying heart condition, and consider inotropic drips such as dobutamine or milrinone.

Notes: _____

Obstructive Shock (Cardiac Tamponade)

This is fluid or blood build-up in pericardial sac surrounding the heart.

- *Causes:* Blunt or penetrating chest trauma.
- *Signs and symptoms:* Penetrating chest wound noted to left third to fifth ribs; dyspnea; facial cyanosis; hypotension; ST-segment elevation in all leads on electrocardiogram; chest wall ecchymosis; and elevated venous pressure. Beck's triad: muffled heart sounds, JVD, and hypotension. Hamman's crunch: crunching, rasping sound heard with the heartbeat.
- *Interventions:* Anticipate orders to monitor cardiac performance, administer oxygen, open IV access, take electrocardiogram, and prepare for emergency pericardiocentesis.

Notes: _____

Question: What autoimmune condition may cause cardiac tamponade?
Answer: *Systemic lupus erythematosus.*

Obstructive Shock (Tension Pneumothorax)

Tension pneumothorax is a life-threatening complication of pneumothorax.

- *Causes:* The lung totally collapses and the heart and chest contents actually shift toward the unaffected lung. Blood flow through the aorta is obstructed as thoracic organs shift to one side.
- *Signs and symptoms:* Tracheal shift; severe respiratory distress; hypotension and JVD; dyspnea; tachypnea; tachycardia; sudden pleuritic chest pain; anxiety; restlessness; asymmetrical chest expansion; diminished or absent breath sounds on affected side; pallor; hypotension if severe; subcutaneous emphysema; and palpitations.
- *Interventions:* Treat ABCs; place in high Fowler's position; anticipate orders to prepare for needle thoracentesis and/or chest tube insertion, administer pain medications, arrange for chest x-ray, and apply sterile nonporous dressing (Vaseline gauze) with tape on three sides over an open, penetrating chest wound.

Notes: _____

Question: When a 27-year-old female arrives in the ED complaining of sudden onset of shortness of breath, what question should you ask?
Answer: *"Are you currently taking any birth control medication?"*

Obstructive Shock Pulmonary Embolus

Pulmonary embolus is a complete or partial thrombus blockage of the pulmonary artery that results in systemic hypoxia.

- *Causes:* Blood clots or air, fat, or amniotic fluid emboli. Risk factors may include history of thrombus or embolism formation, recent surgery, recent travel, estrogen therapy, cancer, postpartum, smoking, and prolonged immobilization.

- *Signs and symptoms:* Sudden dyspnea and tachypnea; respiratory distress; anxiety; restlessness; confusion; chest pain; cough; hemoptysis; wheezing; diaphoresis; pallor from the nipple line up; fever; hypotension; right-sided congestive heart failure, peaked P waves, right bundle branch block (RBBB), ST-segment and T-wave changes on electrocardiogram; JVD; cyanosis; and respiratory arrest.
- *Interventions:* Anticipate orders to give oxygen; obtain pulmonary angiography or pulmonary ventilation/perfusion scan, spiral CT scan; apply bilevel positive airway pressure; use bag valve mask for ventilatory assistance; prepare for intubation; start IV access; administer IV fluids and anticoagulants; use IV or inhaled bronchodilators; and give analgesics, antidysrhythmics, and thrombolytic and platelet aggregation inhibitor therapy.

Notes: _____

Distributive Anaphylactic Shock

Anaphylactic shock is a systemic antigen–antibody response to an allergic reaction that is associated with sudden severe respiratory distress.

- *Causes:* Unknown, but various triggers may stimulate a severe allergic reaction, including seafood, iodine, certain antibiotics, insect bites, nuts, and various medications or food.
- *Signs and symptoms:* Laryngeal edema; bronchospasms; wheezing; angioedema; and hypotension due to peripheral vasodilation.
- *Interventions:* Establish airway; apply oxygen; monitor cardiac performance; open IV access; obtain anaphylactic drug box; and administer medications (epinephrine, antihistamines, bronchodilators, Pepcid, and IV steroid) as ordered.

Notes: _____

Fast Facts in a Nutshell

It is important to understand which concentration of epinephrine to administer for anaphylaxis. You do not want to give the wrong one. As odd as it sounds, an easy way to remember the difference is to compare them to a tequila shot and a margarita. Both drinks have tequila in them, but one is diluted and one is concentrated. Epinephrine also comes in concentrated forms and a diluted form.

- Epinephrine 1:1,000 comes in a 1-mL ampule/vial and is concentrated like a shot of tequila and therefore can be given only subcutaneously or intramuscularly (SQ/IM) for anaphylaxis.
- Epinephrine 1:10,000 comes in a large premixed syringe and is diluted like a margarita. Therefore, it can be given intravenously, typically during cardiopulmonary arrest.
- High-dose epinephrine 1:1,000 contains 30 mL, 30 SQ/ IM doses, or 30 "shots of tequila" in one vial! It is not to be confused with other forms of epinephrine. It is rarely used and no longer indicated in the American Heart Association (AHA) guidelines for advanced cardiopulmonary life support (ACLS).

Distributive Septic Shock

This is a systemic infection or severe sepsis with poor profusion despite adequate fluid resuscitation. The very young, elderly, and immunosuppressed patients are more at risk. It can lead to systemic inflammatory response syndrome (SIRS).

- *Causes:* Typically, due to gram-negative or gram-positive bacteria. The infection usually stems from one source and then spreads to the rest of the body through the bloodstream. A massive inflammatory response is launched by the body, which results in vasodilation and hypotension.
- *Signs and symptoms:* Fever, flushed skin, bounding pulses, vasodilation, tachycardia, widening pulse pressure, and anxiety are noted in early stages. Hypothermia, hypotension, pallor, mottled skin, scant urine output, weakness, and coma are noted in late stages.
- *Interventions:* Look for underlying infection; monitor vital signs and temperature; and anticipate orders to start IV access and fluid bolus of 30 mL/kg (caution if renal failure or congestive heart failure). Obtain blood cultures, complete blood count,

procalcitonin, lactic acid levels; administer IV antibiotics; and obtain urine culture.

Notes: _____

Fast Facts in a Nutshell

SIRS Criteria: Two or more of the following symptoms may be indicative of sepsis:

- Temperature > 38°C (100.4° F) or < 36°C (96.8° F)
- Heart rate > 90 beats per minute
- Respiration rate > 20 breaths per minute, or hyperventilation and $PaCO_2$ < 32 mmHg
- WBC > 12,000 mm^3, < 4,000 mm^3, or > 10% immature neutrophils (bands)

Question: Would you obtain blood cultures before or after administering IV antibiotics?
Answer: *Before. Take cultures from two different sites.*

Distributive Neurogenic Shock

This is the loss of sympathetic vasomotor regulation.

- *Causes:* Brain stem injury, spinal anesthesia, or spinal cord injury. Other causes may include drug use, such as tranquilizers, barbiturates, or anesthetics.
- *Signs and symptoms:* Peripheral vasodilation; neurological deficits; bradycardia, respiratory depression, paraplegia/quadriplegia, priapism, poikilothermia, warm or flushed skin; and severe hypotension.
- *Interventions:* Provide ABCs; maintain cervical (C-spine) immobilization if spinal cord injury is present. Anticipate orders to obtain IV access; administer IV fluid bolus; make neurological assessments; give dopamine or norepinephrine (Levophed), atropine for symptomatic bradycardia; maintain normal temperature; and reduce intracranial pressure.

Notes: _____

Cardiothoracic Traumas

These traumas may be the result of motor vehicle collisions, gunshot wounds, falls, blasts, blows to the chest, or crushing injuries.

Pneumothorax: An air leak in the pleural space resulting in partial or total collapse of the lung.

- *Causes:* A traumatic lung injury or spontaneous rupture that results in an air leak into the pleural space.
- *Signs and symptoms:* Sucking chest wound; dyspnea; tachypnea; tachycardia; sudden pleuritic chest pain; anxiety; restlessness; diminished or absent breath sounds on affected side; pallor; hypotension if severe; subcutaneous emphysema; palpitations; or asymptomatic if small.
- *Interventions:* Put patient in high Fowler's position; give oxygen; cover open chest wounds with flap Vaseline gauze dressing secured on three sides; anticipate orders to check pulse oximetry, connect to cardiac monitor, arrange for immediate chest x-ray, prepare to assist with needle thoracostomy or chest tube insertion, administer pain meds, and obtain IV access.

Notes: _____

Hemothorax: Blood leak in the pleural space resulting in partial or total collapse of the lung.

- *Causes:* Penetrating chest trauma with bleeding into the lung.
- *Signs and symptoms:* If blood loss is greater than 1,500 mL: mediastinal shift (systolic blood pressure of less than 80 mmHg, and capillary refill of more than 4 seconds); decreased urine output; respiratory distress; hypotension; cyanosis; tracheal deviation; decreased or absent breath sounds; and flat neck veins due to hypovolemic shock.
- *Interventions:* Treat ABCs; assist with chest tube insertion; anticipate orders to prepare for emergency thoracotomy, open two large-bore IV accesses, administer IV fluid bolus, monitor cardiac performance, and prepare for emergency blood transfusion. If large volume of blood loss, anticipate autotransfusion.

Notes: _____

Flail chest: Fracture of two or more ribs in two or more places resulting in a free-floating segment of the chest wall. Mortality increases if bilateral injury is present.

- *Causes:* Chest trauma.
- *Signs and symptoms:* Paradoxical chest movement; chest pain; dyspnea; tachypnea; and crepitus.
- *Interventions:* Treat ABCs; anticipate orders to start IV access, monitor pulse oximetry, control pain, and prepare for possible intubation for ventilation assistance.

Notes: _____

> **Question:** What is the most serious injury associated with fractures of first and second ribs?
> **Answer:** *Aortic rupture.*

Ruptured Diaphragm

This is a tear or rupture of the diaphragm; it can be a life-threatening injury.

- *Causes:* Blunt or penetrating forces resulting in herniation of abdominal contents into the thoracic cavity.
- *Signs and symptoms:* Epigastric pain; chest pain; abdominal pain; bowel sounds in lower chest; dyspnea; dysphagia; and decreased breath sounds.
- *Interventions:* Anticipate orders to monitor cardiac performance and pulse oximetry, use nasogastric tube for stomach decompression, establish IV access, and prepare for surgery.

Notes: _____

Spinal Cord Traumas

These traumas may result in spinal shock or neurogenic shock.

- *Causes:* Neck or back trauma.
- *Signs and symptoms:* Breathing difficulty; varying paralysis depending on injury location; bradycardia; hypotension; autonomic dysreflexia (hypertensive condition: headache,

sweating, and bradycardia); warm and dry skin; may assume room temperature; pain; and possible priapism.

- *Interventions:* Open airway maintaining cervical (C-spine) immobilization (use jaw thrust maneuver); conduct a neurological assessment; logroll the patient when turning; prepare for possible endotracheal intubation; assist if ventilation assistance required; anticipate orders to administer IV fluids and steroids, insert nasogastric tube and Foley catheter, provide therapeutic hypothermia per hospital policy, and take measures to avoid skin breakdown.

Notes: _____

Question: Children younger than 8 years of age are most likely to have what type of spinal cord injury?
Answer: *Cervical spine C1 to C3.*

Abdominal Traumas

Splenic injuries: Trauma or injury to the spleen.

- *Causes:* Usually occurs with blunt left upper quadrant abdominal trauma.
- *Signs and symptoms:* Kehr's sign (see Figure 21.1; left upper quadrant abdominal pain that may radiate to the left shoulder); absent or hypoactive bowel sounds; abdominal muscle rigidity; and hypovolemic shock.
- *Interventions:* Frequent abdominal assessments (look, listen, and feel); anticipate orders to establish large-bore IV access; perform focused assessment with sonography in trauma (FAST) ultrasound exam; administer IV fluids, hemoglobin and hematocrit; type and screen blood; and prepare for blood transfusion and surgical intervention. Narrowing pulse pressure may indicate ongoing blood loss.

Notes: _____

Question: In blunt abdominal trauma, which organ is most commonly injured?
Answer: *The spleen.*

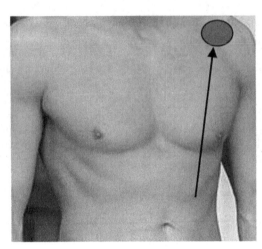

Figure 21.1 Kehr's sign. *Source: Photo by Steve Han (Wikimedia Commons).*

The highly vascular ruptured spleen is a life-threatening injury. Check Kehr's sign (see Figure 21.1), which is a sharp pain radiating to the left scapula.

Pelvic fractures: Either stable or unstable. With a pelvic fracture, your patient can lose up to about 3,000 mL of blood!

- *Causes:* Pelvic trauma.
- *Signs and symptoms:* Pain; pelvic instability; rigidity; hypoactive bowel sounds; hypovolemic shock; and leg shortening or rotation. If urethral laceration: blood from urethral meatus. If bladder laceration: suprapubic pain and an inability to void.
- *Interventions:* Anticipate orders to apply pelvic binder, establish large-bore IV access, administer IV isotonic fluid bolus, arrange for pelvic x-ray or CT scan, type and screen blood, and prepare for possible surgery or interventional radiology.

Notes: _____

Question: What is contraindicated if blood is noted at the urethral meatus?
Answer: *Foley catheter.*

Head Traumas

Linear skull fracture: A nondepressed skull fracture.

- *Causes:* Head trauma.
- *Signs and symptoms:* Pain over fracture; scalp laceration; headache; and possible decreased level of consciousness.
- *Interventions:* Elevate head of bed, obtain neurological assessment; clean and dress any wounds; arrange for skull x-rays or head CT scans; and inform patient of head-injury-patient teaching instructions upon discharge.

Notes: _____

Basilar skull fracture: A fracture to the bones at the base of the skull. Complications include infection and cerebrospinal fluid (CSF) leak.

- *Causes:* Head trauma to base of skull.
- *Signs and symptoms:* Altered level of consciousness; bruising behind the ear (Battle's sign) 12 to 24 hours after injury; bruising around the eyes (Racoon's eyes) 12 to 24 hours after injury; headache; rhinorrhea; otorrhea; and unilateral hearing loss (see Figure 21.2).
- *Interventions:* If there is a CSF leak, apply dry sterile loose dressing below the drainage. Elevate the head of the bed, obtain frequent neurological assessments; anticipate orders to arrange for x-rays and head CT scan, establish IV access, administer antibiotics, and avoid nasogastric tube.

Notes: _____

Depressed skull fracture: A concave-like skull fracture. May be an open fracture; assess for CSF and bleeding.

- *Causes:* Direct blow to the head; head trauma.
- *Signs and symptoms:* Altered level of consciousness; head laceration; headache; and skull depression noted upon palpation.
- *Interventions:* Apply loose sterile dressing; perform frequent neurological assessments; anticipate orders to: establish IV access; administer antibiotics; arrange for operating room admission, x-rays, and head CT scan.

Notes: _____

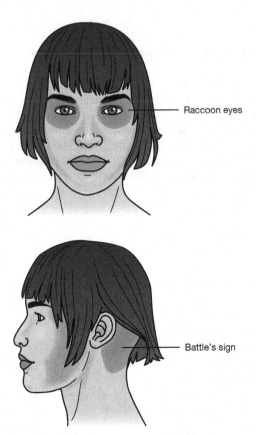

Figure 21.2 Raccoon eyes and Battle's sign.

Fast Facts in a Nutshell

A loose sterile dressing is used on a depressed skull fracture and nasally for rhinorrhea to check for CSF leaks.

Concussion or mild traumatic brain injury: A closed head injury resulting in transient neurological changes with a Glasgow Coma Scale (GCS) of 13 to 15.

- *Causes:* Head trauma.
- *Signs and symptoms:* Nausea; vomiting; dizziness; headache; altered level of consciousness; seizure; poor balance; normal head CT report; and possible amnesia.
- *Interventions:* Perform a neurological assessment; elevate head of bed; anticipate orders for head CT scan and hospital admission if loss of consciousness lasts more than 5 minutes or patient remains confused, and provide head injury discharge instructions. To promote healing and avoid postconcussive or second impact syndromes, sports activities should be restricted until cleared by provider.

Notes: _____

Subdural hematoma: Bleeding between the dura mater (outermost brain covering) and the arachnoid layer (fine fibrous layer between dura and pia mater) of the meninges resulting in direct pressure on brain surface.

- *Causes:* Commonly caused by head trauma or violent shaking.
- *Signs and symptoms:* Loss of consciousness; deteriorating mental status; fixed and dilated pupil on side of injury; increased intracranial pressure; immediate and prolonged coma; and posturing (de**cort**icate, toward the **cor**d; decerebrate, away from the cord; see Figure 21.3).
- *Interventions:* Perform neurological assessment; anticipate orders for a head CT scan, take measures to reduce intracranial pressure, and prepare patient for neurosurgery.

Notes: _____

Epidural hematoma: Bleeding between skull and dura mater.

- *Causes:* Head trauma. This condition commonly occurs with temporal and parietal skull fractures.
- *Signs and symptoms:* Loss of consciousness; ipsilateral pupil dilation; posturing; and hemiparesis.
- *Interventions:* Perform neurological assessment; anticipate orders for a head CT scan, take measures to reduce intracranial pressure, and prepare patient for surgery.

Notes: _____

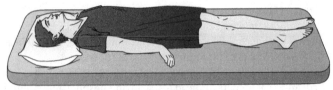

Decerebrate posturing

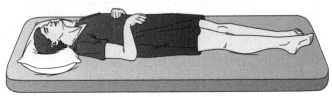

Decorticate posturing

Figure 21.3 Decerebrate and decorticate posturing.

Subarachnoid hemorrhage: Bleeding between pia mater (delicate surface layer of brain) and arachnoid membrane.

- *Causes:* Head trauma. This injury is frequently associated with child abuse and has a high mortality rate.
- *Signs and symptoms:* Headache; nausea and vomiting; altered level of consciousness; neurological deficits; seizure; and posturing.
- *Interventions:* Prepare neurological assessment; anticipate order to arrange for head CT scan; and prepare for surgery.

Notes: _____

Contusion: Bruise to the brain surface.

- *Causes:* Direct blow to the head.
- *Signs and symptoms:* Neurological deficits; altered level of consciousness for more than 6 hours; nausea and vomiting; amnesia; seizure; visual disturbances; and posturing.
- *Interventions:* Perform neurological assessment, immobilize C-spine, arrange for head CT scan when ordered, and provide head-injury-patient teaching upon discharge.

Notes: _____

Increased Intracranial Pressure

- *Causes:* Head trauma, electrolyte imbalances, and meningitis.
- *Signs and symptoms:* Altered level of consciousness; oval-shaped pupil; Cheyne–Stokes respirations; and bulging fontanels in children younger than 2 years of age.
- *Interventions:* Anticipate orders to administer mannitol, administer sedatives, maintain intracranial pressure less than 15 mmHg, elevate head of bed to 30°, and avoid Valsalva maneuver.

Notes: _____

SUMMARY

You now have a stronger knowledge base for shock and multisystem emergencies. Shock and trauma emergencies are always critical situations. You should be able to differentiate among the various types of shock and trauma and know how to respond. Finding time to chart during a critical emergency is difficult. Most of the time, you need another nurse to help. All ED nurses have to be team players. Notify your team and volunteer or ask someone to document as care is provided. Rapid responses save lives and preserve end organs. To ease any anxiety, take some deep and cleansing breaths, get help, and learn as much as you can about shock and trauma.

22

Substance Abuse and Toxicologic Emergencies

Substance abuse and toxicologic conditions, which are seen regularly in the emergency department (ED), can be fatal. Because so many types of substance abuse and poisonous materials exist, remembering them all is difficult. Increasingly, teenagers and young adults are finding creative inexpensive ways to get high. These may include synthetic drugs or household substances such as nutmeg, poisonous flowers, cough syrups, and family members' prescribed home medications. A detailed assessment and patient history is key to identifying the substance taken. Be sure to include feedback from any witnesses, friends, or family who may be willing to disclose what was taken. This chapter provides a simple and easy-to-use substance abuse and toxicology table. Even with access to this table, you must still always consult with poison control after the patient is triaged. Poison control will give you vital individualized suggestions based on the patient's weight, circumstances, amount of drug intake, and the time frame in which the drug was taken. Document and communicate the suggestions provided by poison control with the ED provider to obtain any necessary immediate orders.

During this part of your orientation, locate and become familiar with:

- Local poison control number
- Your local poisonous snakes and appropriate antivenom information
- Nasogastric tubes and gastric lavage equipment
- Medications to know: Charcoal with or without sorbitol, naloxone (Narcan), flumazenil (Romazicon), acetylcysteine (Mucomyst), and banana bag

Fast Facts in a Nutshell

- Call poison control for **every** overdose.
- Treatment of most overdose patients generally begins with the **ABCs** (**A**irway, **B**reathing, **C**irculation) and **MOVE** (**M**onitor, **O**xygen, **V**enous access, and **E**lectrocardiogram).

Table 22.1 is a great quick reference tool to assist you with substance abuse and toxicology cases. In it, you will find an alphabetical list of each substance or drug class, with the corresponding drug-effect symptoms and interventions. Examples of drugs and substances are provided under each class.

Notes: _____

Question: Why can't you rely on a pulse oxygen reading in carbon monoxide poisoning?
Answer: *Carbon dioxide, ethane, methane, propane, and other fuel gases bind to hemoglobin, preventing oxygen from binding to the hemoglobin. Therefore, you cannot rely on a pulse oxygen reading. Treatment is "fresh air" or supplemental oxygen.*

Question: Ecstasy use along with increased water intake to avoid hyperthermia can lead to what electrolyte imbalance?
Answer: *Hyponatremia.*

Question: A college student arrives in the ED complaining of palpitations and chest pain. He admits to using cocaine. What should you suspect?
Answer: *Acute myocardial infarction.*

Question: How does charcoal leave the digestive system?
Answer: *Usually it comes out in the form of black diarrhea. An unconscious or confused patient may need an incontinence pad.*

Table 22.1

Substance Abuse and Toxicology Table		
Drug/substance	Signs and symptoms	Interventions/anticipated orders
Acetylcholinesterase inhibition (cholinergics) Insecticides, organophosphates, carbamates, and nerve agents	Remember **SLUDGE:** Saliva, Lacrimation, Urination, Defecation, GI (gastrointestinal) upset, and Emesis. Early on tachycardia; lethargic; paralysis; shock; anxiety; bronchospasms; ataxia; pulmonary edema; bradypnea; seizure; and coma. Bradycardia in late stages	Wash toxins off the patient. If oral ingestion, give 1 g/kg charcoal. Atropine may reverse central nervous system effects. Ipratropium bromide (Atrovent) nebulized treatment may dry secretions. Administer pralidoxime or obidoxime as ordered
Alcohol abuse Liquors, beers, wines, moonshine, rubbing alcohol, even mouthwash	Slurred speech; unsteady gait; and alcohol odor. The patient may go into withdrawal	Obtain alcohol level. Intravenous (IV) banana bag and time for alcohol levels to drop. Lorazepam (Ativan) helps with withdrawal

(continued)

Table 22.1

Substance Abuse and Toxicology Table *(continued)*

Drug/substance	Signs and symptoms	Interventions/anticipated orders
Anticholinergic overdose Dicyclomine, tropicamide, alkaloids cyclopentolate, homatropine, phenothiazines, amanita muscarina, jimson-weed or deadly nightshade, belladonna, atropine, and tricyclics	Hallucinations; delirium; blurred vision; tachycardia; arrhythmias; fever; abdominal distention; urine retention; ataxia; cardiovascular collapse; seizure; hypertension; thirst; hot/flushed/dry skin; dilated pupils; and mydriasis	Physostigmine and 1 g/kg charcoal if ingestion was less than 1 hour ago
Benzodiazepines Serax, Rohypnol aka "roofies" are 10 times as potent as diazepam	Drowsiness; confusion; bradypnea; sedation; and hypotension	Administer flumazenil (Romazicon). May cause seizures. Caution if unknown ingestion and consider seizure precautions
Beta-blockers Atenolol, metoprolol, propranolol, and sotalol	Bradycardia; hypotension; shock; and cardiac arrest	Administer 1–5 mg gluconate intravenously/intramuscularly/subcutaneously. Atropine for symptomatic bradycardia. Give IV normal saline bolus for hypotension; and prepare pacemaker and calcium IV push
Calcium channel blockers Verapamil, nifedipine (Procardia), and diltiazem	Bradycardia; hypotension; lethargy; confusion; bradypnea; nausea and vomiting; shock; hyperglycemia; and cardiac arrest	1 g calcium gluconate or calcium chloride intravenously over 5 minutes until response seen or maximum of 4 g. Give normal saline bolus

(continued)

Table 22.1

Substance Abuse and Toxicology Table *(continued)*

Drug/substance	Signs and symptoms	Interventions/anticipated orders
Carbon monoxide poisoning Carbon monoxide displaces oxygen on the hemoglobin	Hypoxia; confusion; headache; nausea and vomiting; dizziness; coma; seizures; cyanosis; and death	Give oxygen via nonrebreather mask; provide hyperbaric oxygen treatment; and obtain carbon dioxide levels
Cardiac glycosides Digoxin, digitoxin, oleander, and foxglove	Visual yellow-green halos; nausea and vomiting; headache; bradycardia; ventricular arrhythmias; shock; and cardiac arrest	Obtain digoxin level; give digoxin (Digibind) immune fab; administer 1 g/kg charcoal and 1 mg/kg lidocaine intravenously for arrhythmias, and give atropine
Ethylene glycol (antifreeze)	First 1–12 hours: slurred speech; inebriated; coma; seizure; and death. 12–24 hours: tachycardia; hypertension; tachypnea; congestive heart failure; acute respiratory distress syndrome; and cardiac collapse. 24–72 hours: nephrotoxicity; flank pain; renal failure; and hypocalcemia	Labs: determine serum ethylene glycol level; prepare basic metabolic panel; and obtain urinalysis. Give gastric lavage (charcoal is ineffective), 50 mEq IV sodium bicarbonate; 10% 10–20 mL calcium gluconate intravenously, 2 g IV magnesium; 100 mg IV thiamine; 15 mg/kg IV fomepizole (Antizol); and prepare for dialysis
Hallucinogens LSD (D-lysergic acid diethylamide) abuse	Agitation; hallucinations; dilated pupils; hyperthermic; and tachycardia	Reassure and reorient to reality; instruct patient to keep eyes open; and provide good lighting to decrease shadows. Give benzodiazepines for agitation

(continued)

Table 22.1

Substance Abuse and Toxicology Table *(continued)*

Drug/substance	Signs and symptoms	Interventions/anticipated orders
Ibuprofen, nonsteroidal anti-inflammatory drugs (NSAIDs)	Nausea; vomiting; abdominal pain; drowsiness; tarry or bloody stools; hemoptysis; shallow breathing; syncope; or coma	Activated charcoal within 1–4 hours postingestion; supportive care; maintain airway, breathing, and circulation (ABCs); gastric lavage if acute ingestion of massive amounts; hemodialysis to correct acidosis; benzodiazepines for seizures
Heparin	Bleeding	Obtain partial thromboplastin time level and give protamine sulfate
Insulin	Weakness; lethargic; syncope; and blood sugar less than 80	Monitor blood sugar; give 1-amp dextrose (D50) intravenously, if alert feed the patient a meal; give intramuscular (IM) glucagon as ordered if IV access unobtainable
Iron	Initially: hypotension; nausea; vomiting; and bloody stools. Late (2–3 days): coagulopathies; metabolic acidosis; hemorrhage; renal failure; liver failure; and shock	Deferoxamien mesylate (Desferal) binds with iron and is excreted via the kidneys

(continued)

Table 22.1

Substance Abuse and Toxicology Table *(continued)*

Drug/substance	Signs and symptoms	Interventions/anticipated orders
3,4-methylenedioxy-methamphetamine (MDMA) Ecstasy, Molly	Euphoria; increased trust; tachycardia; hypertension; hyperthermia; sweating; muscle cramps; sexual arousal; chills; depression; and blurred vision	Treatment is supportive. Treat ABCs first. Cooling blanket or device may be ordered to regulate temperature. IV fluids may be ordered to treat electrolyte imbalances (hyponatremia). Consider activated charcoal if recent ingestion.
Nonspecific or unknown	Varies. Complete a thorough assessment and patient history for any clues	Treat symptoms. Consider activated charcoal in water or 1 g/kg sorbitol.
Narcotics (opioids) Morphine, methadone, dextromethorphan, heroin, fentanyl, meperidine (Demerol), codeine, diphenoxylate and propoxyphene	Pinpoint pupils (miosis); central nervous system depression; depression; bradycardia; hypotension; and bradypnea	IV 0.4–2 mg naloxone (Narcan) every 2–3 minutes up to 10 mg
Neuroleptics Metroclopramide, haloperidol, thioxanthenes, and phenothiazines	EKG changes (prolonged Q-T segments); dysrhythmias; and altered level of consciousness	Benzotropine (Congentin) blocks dopamine reuptake
Salicylates Aspirin	Nausea and vomiting; tinnitus; diaphoresis; acidosis; altered mental status; seizures; and shock	Dialysis and 1 mEq/kg sodium bicarbonate intravenously

(continued)

Table 22.1

Substance Abuse and Toxicology Table *(continued)*

Drug/substance	Signs and symptoms	Interventions/anticipated orders
Stimulants (sympathomimetics) Aminophylline, amphetamines, cocaine, ephedrine, caffeine, methylphenidates, methamphetamines, and phencyclidine (PCP)	Hypertension; dilated pupils; tachycardia; paranoia; vasoconstriction; hyperthermia; seizures; chest pain; acute myocardial infarction; coma (hypotension with caffeine); and altered mood	Give benzodiazepines, nitroglycerin or nitroprusside (Nipride) for hypertension, haloperidol (Haldol), and 1 g/kg charcoal
Synthetic cannabinoids New psychoactive substances (NPS), synthetic marijuana, K-2, or Spice	Relaxation; euphoria; anxiety; tachycardia; hypertension; diaphoresis; delusions; paranoia; psychosis; hallucinations; seizures; nausea and vomiting; and aggressive or violent behavior toward self or others. May lead to renal failure	Antidotes and routine toxicology screening for synthetic cannabinoids are currently unavailable. Treatment is supportive. Benzodiazepines may be ordered for agitation or seizures. Antiemetics may be ordered for nausea. IV fluids may be ordered to correct any electrolyte imbalances.
Synthetic cathinones Bath salts, alpha-pyrrolidinopentiophenone (alpha-PVP) (Flakka)	Stimulant effects; sweating; palpitations; hallucinations; paranoid; pyschosis; aggressive violent behavior toward self or others; anxiety; agitation; hyperthermia; hypertension can lead to renal failure or myocardial infarction	Antidotes and routine toxicology screening for synthetic cathinones are currently unavailable. Treatment is supportive. Benzodiazepines can help with agitation and seizures. Restraints may be ordered for safety. Antipsychotics may be given with caution as they tend to lower seizure thresholds.

(continued)

Table 22.1

Substance Abuse and Toxicology Table *(continued)*

Drug/substance	Signs and symptoms	Interventions/anticipated orders
Tricyclic antidepressants Amitriptyline, desipramine, nortriptyline, and imipramine	Tachycardia; nausea; vomiting; tachydysrhythmias; hypotension; seizures; shock; and cardiac arrest	Give IV sodium bicarbonate for tricyclic antidepressants to obtain serum pH of 7.50–7.55 to alter protein binding; give normal saline bolus; give isotonic fluids and norepinephrine (Levophed) if hypotensive; and consider activated charcoal
Tylenol overdose Can lead to liver failure and death. Toxic doses destroy hepatocytes resulting in liver damage and necrosis. 140 mg/kg is toxic	First 24 hours: asymptomatic; minor gastrointestinal upset. 24–72 hours: elevated liver function test or renal failure. 72–96 hours: jaundice; renal failure; coagulopathy; and liver necrosis. 4 days–2 weeks: symptoms resolve or patient dies	Labs: acetaminophen level 4 hours after ingestion. Administer *N*-acetylcysteine (Mucomyst), the sooner the better; may be useful up to 72 hours after ingestion
Venom of rattlesnakes, cotton mouths, and copperheads	Bite/fang marks with redness/ bruising; pain; and swelling	Antivenom, crotalidae polyvalent (CroFab) three to five vials in 250–500 mg normal saline for mild symptoms
Warfarin (Coumadin)	Bleeding	Obtain prothrombin time and international normalized ratio (INR) level, and give phytonadione (vitamin K)

SUMMARY

You now have a stronger knowledge base for substance abuse and toxicology emergencies. You should be able to differentiate the types of substance abuse and toxicology emergencies and know how to respond. It is vital to obtain the best history possible from your patient. Because your patient may not be responsive, speak with any witnesses, friends, or family. Each overdose case is different. Many factors will affect the treatment, including time of ingestion, amount of substance, patient's weight, and current vital signs. Be sure to contact poison control for every case. They will help you and the provider come up with the proper individualized treatment course needed.

23

Triage

Although most emergency departments (EDs) have a triage area, triage is not actually a place, but a process. If you think about it, you can triage a patient anywhere, even in the parking lot! By definition, triage is a French-derived word that means "to choose or to sort." Sorting sounds simple enough. So what is the big deal? Well, the decisions made by the triage nurse determine the level of care and urgency in which a patient will be seen. For instance, say you triage a 21-year-old female with severe right-sided abdominal pain as a level 3 or nonurgent. You think to yourself, "She is not that sick because she looks fine." She waits several hours while all the level 2 or urgent patients are seen by the doctor. When the doctor finally sees her, she is now hypotensive and bleeding internally because her ectopic pregnancy has ruptured. As you can see, the decisions made in triage can directly affect patient outcomes. It sounds scary, but with the right training, experience, and critical thinking skills, you too can master the art of triage. This chapter provides you with some of the tools you will need. After studying this chapter, you should be able to identify which patients can wait and which patients cannot wait, differentiate the levels of triage acuity, perform an across-the-room assessment, and list the common pitfalls of triage.

During this part of your orientation, locate and become familiar with:

- Your facility's triage acuity system and documentation requirements
- Your ED's triage protocol orders

(continued)

- Pediatric vital signs
- Your facility's policy on isolation and infection control
- Emergency Medical Treatment and Labor Act (EMTALA)
- Security notification and panic buttons
- The patient liaison or representative
- Your facility's lockdown procedure and policy
- Your facility's "left without being seen" policy
- Location of ice packs, dressings, and triage medication supplies

BEFORE YOU CAN TRIAGE

Not just anyone can be a triage nurse. The weight of the decisions made by the triage nurse is heavy. These decisions require sound critical thinking skills, a strong nursing foundation, the ability to multitask, and excellent interpersonal skills. Most EDs require a triage nurse to have a certain amount of experience, specific certifications, and evidence of having taken a triage class or competency. The Emergency Nurses Association (ENA) recommends triage be conducted by a registered nurse who has received formal triage training and holds the following certifications: Cardiopulmonary Resuscitation (CPR), Advanced Cardiac Life Support (ACLS), Emergency Nurse Pediatric Course (ENPC), Trauma Nurse Core Course (TNCC), Geriatric Emergency Nursing Education (GENE), and Board Certified Emergency Nurse (BCEN). Take the initiative to find out what competencies are required and what triage classes are available at your facility and sign up for them.

TRIAGE ACUITY SYSTEMS

Believe it or not, there are a variety of triage acuity systems. While your ED may use a five-level triage acuity system, one of the neighboring EDs may be using a three-level triage acuity system. The first thing you must do is identify the triage system your ED is using. Table 23.1 demonstrates some of the differences among the various systems.

EMERGENCY SEVERITY INDEX

Although there are many different triage systems, the latest research conducted by the ENA supports the use of a five-level system such as

Table 23.1

Level	Five-level systems	Four-level systems	Three-level systems	Two-level systems
Comparing Triage Systems				
1	Resuscitation	Life-threatening		
2	Emergent	Emergent	Emergent	Emergent
3	Urgent	Urgent	Urgent	
4	Nonurgent	Nonurgent	Nonurgent	Nonemergent
5	Referred			

Level 1 or resuscitation: Requires immediate life-saving interventions.

Level 2 or emergent: A high-risk situation, confused/lethargic/disoriented patient, in severe pain or distress, or has dangerously abnormal vital signs.

Level 3 or urgent: Requires many resources.

Level 4 or nonurgent: Requires just one resource.

Level 5 or referred: Requires no resources.

the Emergency Severity Index (ESI). Similar five-level triage scales include the Canadian Triage and Acuity Scale, Australasian Triage Scale, and the Manchester Triage System.

Fast Facts in a Nutshell

ESI level is determined by answering four simple questions:

- Is the patient dying or in need of life-saving interventions?
- Is this a patient who will deteriorate if he or she is placed in the waiting room?
- How many resources are needed?
- What are the vital signs?

RESOURCES

The next question you may be asking is, "What exactly is a resource?" Resources consist of labs, CT, x-ray, MRI, specialty consults, simple procedures, intravenous fluids or medications, intramuscular medications, and inhaled medications. Complex procedures such as moderate sedation count as two resources. However, do not be fooled! There are some interventions that do *not* actually count as a resource. These include intravenous access, pelvic exam, point-of-care testing, consult to the patient's primary physician, simple dressings, slings, crutches, and splints.

CHOOSING AN ACUITY LEVEL

Now that you know which triage system your facility is using, you will need specific information to select the appropriate acuity level. First you will need an "across-the-room" assessment, followed by a chief complaint, interview with patient, vital signs, and focused physical exam.

- *Across-the-room assessment:* This is exactly as it reads. What do you see when you look across the room as the patient approaches the triage desk? In order to do this well, the triage nurse must be in a position to view the entire waiting room. Things to look for include the following:
  - General appearance: Alert or unresponsive, crying, laughing, talking, any obvious deformities, or bloody clothing.
  - Work of breathing: Labored or unlabored, coughing, drooling, gasping, wheezing, rapid or slow respiratory rate, or use of accessory muscles.
  - Circulation: Pink or pale, diaphoretic, flushed, normal, or jaundice.

Fast Facts in a Nutshell

If you find an unstable patient entering the waiting room, do not delay care. If he or she is unstable, bypass the triage area altogether and take the patient to a bed to begin treatment. For example: If a family member wheels a pale, diaphoretic, unresponsive patient into the waiting room, do *not* stop to take vital signs and interview the patient! The patient is unresponsive. Bring the patient back for treatment immediately. Remember, triage is a process, not a place; it can be done in the back simultaneously as the patient receives care.

- *Elicit chief complaint:* The first question to ask is, "What brought you in to see us today?" Certain chief complaints can carry higher risks than others. For example, chest pain would be a higher risk chief complaint than toe injury. The patient with chest pain could be having a fatal heart attack, whereas toe injuries, though painful, are not usually fatal.
- *Interview the patient:* Triage is not the time to conduct an entire head-to-toe assessment. Your goal in triage is to elicit the essential facts needed to make an acuity decision. You should be asking questions that relate to the chief complaint. Look over the triage document at your facility. Most ED triage screening tools include the following:
  - Duration of the chief complaint
  - Related symptoms
  - Mechanism of injury
  - Medical history
  - Current medications (prescription or nonprescription)
  - Immunizations
  - Last menstrual period
  - Allergies
  - Height and weight
  - Department-specific screening questions
- *Obtain vital signs:* Vital signs can influence your final acuity section. If the patient looks fine, has a normal exam, and tells you, "I just feel dizzy," you might not think too much of it. But once you take the patient's blood pressure and it is 289/132, you will think differently. Be sure to memorize the different age-specific normal average vital signs shown in Table 23.2.
- *Conduct a focused physical assessment:* Now that you have collected your subjective data (what the patient says), it is time to document what you see (objective data). If the patient tells you, "I twisted my ankle," take off his socks and shoes and document what the ankle looks like: swollen, obviously deformed, bruised, edematous? Is it tender upon palpation? Are distal pulses present? Is the patient ambulatory?

TRIAGE INTEVENTIONS

Triage simply means to sort, but at times you will need to implement some basic interventions. These interventions may include basic life support, cervical immobilization, isolation procedures,

Table 23.2

Age-Specific Normal Vital Signs

Age	Newborn	Infant	Toddler	Preschooler	School age	Adolescent	Adult
Respirations	40–60	30–63	22–37	20–28	18–25	12–20	12–20
Heart rate	90–205	90–180	80–140	65–120	58–115	50–100	60–100
Systolic blood pressure	67–84	72–104	86–106	89–112	97–115	110–131	120

some medications (e.g., aspirin for chest pain), electrocardiogram (should precede the triage of a chest pain patient), point-of-care blood glucose, and simple wound care (e.g., splinting or ice packs).

- The entire triage process should only take about 2 to 5 minutes. Do not be discouraged at first. Speed and efficiency come with time and practice. Learning to multitask will help. For example, you can apply the blood pressure cuff and pulse oximeter to collect vital signs while interviewing the patient.
- Triage documentation is a legal document and should support your acuity decision. Document both subjective and objective data, behaviors, and quotes when applicable. Do *not* document judgments.
- Always accurately weigh pediatric patients; their medications are based on their *current* weight.

Pediatrics

Triaging pediatric patients can be quite different than triaging adults. Treat the patient and the family as one unit. Typically, it is best to start with the least invasive assessment and interventions to the most invasive. For example, a rectal temperature may cause the infant to cry interfering with observational assessments. Provide honest answers with kid-friendly words. Be familiar with the normal vital signs for each age group. Obtain actual weights. Remember that fevers without an obvious infection source will require multiple resources. In addition, any petechial or purpuric rashes, especially with mental status changes, are a red flag for meningitis or septic shock.

Emergency Medical Treatment and Labor Act (EMTALA)

If you are the triage nurse, "hospitality" is your middle name! By law, you cannot turn any patient away or even discourage him or her from seeking emergency medical care. The EMTALA is known as the federal "anti-dumping" law. It was enacted in 1986 to prohibit hospitals from refusing to see or transfer financially "undesirable." Prior to this law, patients died in the back of ambulances driving from hospital to hospital, seeking an accepting facility. Under EMTALA, hospitals are obligated to provide a nondiscriminatory medically screening exam to any patient seeking care within 250 yards of the hospital. **Understand that a triage assessment is not typically the same as a medical screening exam unless a provider is at triage**. If a medical emergency condition exists, the hospital is obligated to provide stabilizing interventions. Failure to uphold this law can result in a fine of up to $50,000.

COMMON PITFALLS OF TRIAGE

Once you spend a little time in triage you might say to yourself, "Oh, this is not so hard, I've got this." But tread carefully; even the most experienced ED nurse can be fooled. Following is a list of everyday chief complaints or issues that at first glance appear simple or vague. However, in reality, these might actually be much more emergent than they appear. In triage you must always assume the worst-case scenario, and ask questions to rule out that "worst-case" possibility:

- "I feel weak" or "I am dizzy."
    - *What you might be thinking*: This is a very vague complaint. It could just be the flu, a virus, heat exhaustion, or a fever.
    - *What you should be thinking*: What are the worst things that could make someone feel weak or dizzy? Hypoglycemia, hyperglycemia, dehydration, hypotension or hypertension, hypoxia, sepsis, myocardial infarction, stroke, and arrhythmias.
- "I have a headache."
    - *What you might be thinking*: So do I. The patient just wants pain medication.
    - *What you should be thinking*: What is the worst thing this could be? Hypertension, meningitis, cerebral bleed, brain tumor, head injury, concussion. What is the patient's neurological status? What is his or her blood pressure?
- The patient does not look very sick.
    - *What you might be thinking*: If the patient looks fine, it cannot be that bad.
    - *What you should be thinking*: Legally, your opinion does not matter. Look at your subjective and objective data. Is this a high-risk situation?

I once triaged a 73-year-old female having chest pain who "looked fine to me." She was pink, warm, and dry with normal vital signs. She was not clutching her chest, had no previous medical problems, and did not take any medications. She appeared otherwise "healthy." Although I chose the correct acuity level for her, she still surprised me. When we did the EKG, she was having an ST-segment elevated myocardial infarction or STEMI. In laymen's terms, she was "having the big one!" She did not display the typical diaphoretic, anxious, and "there is an elephant on my chest" symptoms. Because I chose the correct acuity level, she received timely appropriate care, despite my opinion that she looked fine.

- "I fell."
    - *What you might be thinking*: Treat the injury. If the bleeding is controlled, everything is okay. Ground-level falls are not dangerous.
    - *What you should be thinking*: Why did the patient fall? Hypoglycemia, stroke, hypotension, medication, or arrhythmia. Was the patient dizzy or weak before the fall, or did she trip and fall? Is a head or C-spine injury involved? Is the patient on anticoagulants? Did the patient lose consciousness? What is the neurological status? Did the patient consume any alcohol or drugs beforehand? Does the patient have a heart condition?
- "My doctor told me to come here."
    - *What you might be thinking*: Those primary care doctors send all their patients here because they do not have time to see them today. If it was serious they would have called an ambulance or gone to another hospital.
    - *What you should be thinking*: What is the phone number to the primary physician? What tests were performed at the office? What symptoms made the patient call his doctor today? Some patients go to the doctor when they should come to the ED.
- The patient is not telling you the whole story.
    - *What you might be thinking*: "This does not make any sense." The symptoms do not align with what the patient is saying.
    - *What you should be thinking*: What is the patient's neurological status? Why does this person think he cannot tell me what is really wrong? Did the patient consume any alcohol or drugs? Does he think you will call the police? Perhaps he thinks insurance won't pay, or he may be too embarrassed.

- "I feel anxious."
  - *What you might be thinking*: Oh, she has a history of panic attacks; it's just a panic attack. This patient is just being dramatic.
  - *What you should be thinking*: Anxious people get sick too! Has the patient ever felt quite like this before? Hypoxia, anaphylaxis, cardiac event, cerebrovascular accident, even things that are very painful such as bowel obstruction or kidney stones can cause a person to appear "anxious."
- "I have back pain."
  - *What you might be thinking*: Another patient with back pain! They just want pain medication.
  - *What you should be thinking*: Kidney stones, shingles, pyelonephritis, dissecting renal or thoracic aneurysm, or is there a spinal injury? Has the patient lost control of his bowels or bladder? Does the pain radiate to the groin or leg? Are there any urinary problems? Is paralysis noted on assessment? Did the pain occur suddenly or gradually?
- "I have been vomiting."
  - *What you might be thinking:* They just need some Zofran and ginger ale and they can go home. It is just another stomach flu.
  - *What you should be thinking*: What is the worst-case scenario of what this could be? Diabetic ketoacidosis, chemotherapy, bowel obstruction, increased intracranial pressure, cardiac problem, food poisoning, or pregnancy. Consider how many times the patient vomited. What is the result of too much vomiting? Electrolyte imbalance and dehydration.

SUMMARY

After reading this chapter, you will gain some of the tools necessary to triage effectively. When used properly, your new triage skills provide communication of care needed across the entire ED. With practice, your triage skills will improve and you will easily identify which patients can wait and which patients cannot wait, differentiate the levels of triage acuity, perform an across-the-room assessment, and list the common pitfalls of triage. Be sure to review your facility's triage requirements and policies. Although you may not qualify to triage for some time, you may find it helpful to observe the triage operation and process during your orientation.

Appendices

Appendix A
Common Emergency Department Lab Values

Lab	Normal value	High-value causes	Low-value causes
Alanine aminotransferase/ serum glutamic pyruvic transaminase (ALT/SGPT)	30–65	Liver damage	
Amylase	25–115	Pancreatitis; cholecystitis	
Anion gap	<11	Diabetic ketoacidosis (DKA)	
Aspartate aminotransferase/serum glutamic-oxaloacetic transaminase (AST/ SGOT)	15–37	Liver damage	Insulin overdose
Beta-hydroxybutyrate	<0.4	Diabetic ketoacidosis	
Blood urea nitrogen (BUN)	7–18	Renal disease	

(*continued*)

Lab	Normal value	High-value causes	Low-value causes
Brain-type natriuretic peptide (BNP) and NT proBNP	Varies by gender and age BNP <100 NT proBNP <300	Right-sided heart failure; pulmonary hypertension; acute pulmonary embolism; or acute coronary syndromes	
Calcium (Ca)	8.5–10.6	Hyperthyroidism; tuberculosis; too much vitamin D	Pancreatitis; parathyroid trauma; alcohol abuse; renal failure
Carboxyhemoglobin level	<1.5%	Carbon monoxide poisoning	
Creatine kinase-MB (CKMB)	0–3.6	Myocardial infarction	
Creatinine	0.6–1.3	Renal disease	
D-dimer	0–682	Congestive heart failure; pulmonary embolism	
Hematocrit (HCT)	37–47	Dehydration	Anemia; gastrointestinal bleeding
Hemoglobin (HGB)	12–16	Dehydration	Anemia; gastrointestinal bleeding
Lactic acid	4.5–19.8	Oxygen deprivation and sepsis	
Lipase	114–286	Pancreatitis; cholecystitis	

(continued)

Lab	Normal value	High-value causes	Low-value causes
Partial thromboplastin time (PTT)	18–41 (varies)	Hemophilia; heparin overdose; disseminated intravascular coagulation (DIC)	
Platelets (PLT)	140–440	Chronic inflammation	Thrombocyto-penia
Potassium (K) CO_2	3.5–5.1 21–32	Metabolic acidosis; respiratory acidosis	Poor potassium intake; diuretics; nausea, vomiting, and diarrhea
Procalcitonin (PCT)	<0.15	Systemic bacterial infection; sepsis	
Prothrombin time (PT)	11–14 (varies)	Coumadin overdose; decreased potassium; liver disease	
Red blood cell (RBC) count	4.2–5.5	Dehydration	Anemia
Sodium (Na)	135–145	Sweating; diarrhea; diabetes	Congestive heart failure; cirrhosis; renal failure; nausea, vomiting, and diarrhea; excess water intake
Troponin	0–0.10	Myocardial infarction	
White blood cell count (WBC)	4–11	Infection; inflammation; leukemia—very high levels	Neutropenia

Appendix B
Everyday Emergency
Department Medications[a]

Medication	Dose	Use
Acetaminophen (Tylenol®, Datril®)	Adult: 650 to 1,000 mg Max dose: 3,000 to 4,000 mg/d Children: 10 to 15 mg/kg; do *not* exceed five doses in 24 hours; max dose 75 mg/kg/d Not to exceed 3,000 to 4,000 mg/d	Fever and analgesic
Acetaminophen with codeine (Tylenol with codeine)	Doses vary Codeine component of 15 to 60 mg. Every 4 hours PO as needed for pain Children: Codeine 0.5 to 1 mg/kg/dose every 4 to 6 hours PO as needed for pain; max dose = 60 mg Refer to acetaminophen dosing section.	Opioid analgesic Suspension: acetaminophen 120 mg and codeine 12 mg per 5 mL

(*continued*)

Medication	Dose	Use
Acetylcysteine (Acetadote®, Mucomyst®)	Adult/children: Oral 72-hour regimen: Loading dose: 140 mg/kg × 1 Maintenance dose: 70 mg/kg every 4 hours × 17 doses; repeat dose if emesis occurs within 1 hour of administration. Acetadote IV 21-hour regimen: Loading dose: 150 mg/kg (max: 15 g) infused over 1 hour Second dose: 50 mg/kg (max: 5 g) infused over 4 hours Third dose: 100 mg/kg (max: 10 g) infused over 16 hours	Antidote for acetaminophen (Tylenol) overdose
Acetylsalicylic acid (aspirin)	75 to 325 mg by mouth or by rectum; indication determines dosing interval	Antiplatelet, analgesic, NSAID
Adenosine (Adenocard®)	Initial 6 mg rapid IV push over 1 to 2 seconds. Follow with 20 mL normal saline bolus. Second dose of 12 mg rapid IV push. Children <50 kg: initial 0.05 to 0.1 mg/kg rapid IV push dose. Second dose 0.1 to 0.2 mg/kg. Children ≥50 kg refer to adult dosing.	Narrow complex PSVT or SVT; *Not* for A-fib, A-flutter, or VT
Albuterol (Proventil®, Ventolin®, Proair®)	Children: Metered dose inhaler (MDI) 90 mcg/puff; four to eight puffs every 20 minutes for three doses, then every 1 to 4 hours as needed; nebulizer: 0.1 to 0.15 mg/kg/dose every 20 minutes for three doses, then 0.15 to 3 mg/kg (max: 10 mg) every 1 to 4 hours as needed. Adult: MDI; four to eight puffs every 20 minutes for up to 4 hours, then every 1 to 4 hours as needed; nebulizer: 2.5 to 5 mg every 20 minutes for three doses, then 2.5 to 10 mg every 1 to 4 hours or 10 to 15 mg/hr continuous.	Bronchodilator for asthma/chronic obstructive pulmonary disease. Also treat hyperkalemia

(continued)

Medication	Dose	Use
Alteplase (Activase®)	Wt based dosing refer to hospital protocol	Thrombolytic (clot buster); acute ischemic stroke, massive pulmonary embolism, and STEMI
Amiodarone hydrochloride (Cordarone®, Nexterone®, Pacerone®)	150 mg IV over 10 minutes, then 1 mg/min IV for 6 hours, followed by 0.5 mg/min for 18 hours Pulseless VT or VF: 300 mg IV push, second dose 150 mg IV push	Life-threatening ventricular arrhythmias
Atropine sulfate (Atropen®)	IV push: 0.5 to 1 mg every 3 to 5 minutes. Maximum of 3 mg. ET: 2 to 3 mg in 10 mL normal saline	Symptomatic bradycardia. For organophosphate poisoning, use 2 mg Atropen.
Azithromycin (Zithromax®)	Adult outpatient pneumonia 500 mg first dose, then 250 mg every day for 4 days. For Chlamydia 1 g PO for one dose IV: 500 mg/d	Antibiotic commonly used for Chlamydia; PID; and respiratory infections.
Banana Bag (1 L D_5 NS or NS, 1 mg folic acid, 10 mL MVI, and 100 mg thiamine) ±1 to 3 g magnesium sulfate	100 to 250 mL/hr IV	Chronic alcohol abuse and malnourishment
Calcium chloride	200 to 1,000 mg IV slowly 100 mg/min or 45 to 90 mg/kg/hr in nonemergent situations. Do *not* mix with sodium bicarbonate or phosphate containing solutions. Central line preferred	Hyperkalemia, calcium channel or beta-blocker overdose, hypocalcemia, and magnesium toxicity

(*continued*)

Medication	Dose	Use
Calcium gluconate	One-third potency of calcium chloride 1,000 mg to 2,000 mg; do *not* mix with sodium bicarbonate or phosphate containing solutions; may be administered peripherally	Hyperkalemia, calcium channel or beta-blocker overdose, hypocalcemia, and magnesium toxicity
Ceftriaxone sodium (Rocephin®). *For IM can mix with lidocaine 1% as directed on box*	Adult: 250 mg to 2 g IV or IM every 12 to 24 hours. Children: 25 to 50 mg/kg/ every 12 hours	Antibiotic for infection
Charcoal in water. No sorbitol for a child due to diarrhea/ dehydration	Infants <1 year: 10 to 25 g Children 1 to 12 years: 25 to 50 g Children >12 years/adults: Initial dose 50 to 100 g, then 25 to 50 g every 4 hours	Antidote for toxins. Can mix with chocolate syrup, Coke, or fruit juice for children.
Charcoal with sorbitol	Adult: Refer to charcoal dosing section.	Antidote for toxins
$D_{50}W$, glucose (dextrose)	Average dose 0.5 to 1 amp intravenous. Check blood sugar.	Acute hypoglycemia; *Use D25 for children.*
Diazepam (Valium®). *Do not mix with anything*	IV: 2 to 10 mg. Per rectum: 0.2 mg/kg (max: 30 mg)	Seizures and sedation
Digoxin (Lanoxin®)	Loading: 0.25 mg to 0.6 mg PO or IV	A-fib, A-flutter, heart failure, or SVT
Digoxin immune Fab (Digibind®)	Varies depending on digoxin level, with an average 400 to 800 mg	Digoxin overdose; digitalis toxicity
Diltiazem hydrochloride (Cardizem®)	20 mg (0.25 mg/kg) IV over 2 minutes. May repeat in 15 minutes at 0.35 mg/kg. Continuous infusion: 5 to 15 mg/hr	A-fib or A-flutter

(*continued*)

Medication	Dose	Use
Dobutamine (Dobutrex®)	IV dose: 2.5 to 40 mcg/kg/min 2.5 to 20 mcg/kg/min IV for postcardiac arrest	Vasopressor. Pump problems: congestive heart failure without symptoms of shock
Dopamine hydrochloride (Intropin®)	IV dose: 5 to 20 mcg/kg/min. May titrate drip in 5 to 10 mcg/kg/min increments	Vasopressor for symptomatic bradycardia, hypotension, or shock
Enalapril maleate (Vasotec®) Enalaprilat (IV formulation)	2.5 to 40 mg PO daily; IV: 1.25 mg/dose over 5 min every 6 hours as needed	Hypertension
Enoxaparin (Lovenox®)	0.75 to 1 mg/kg twice daily dependent on indication; subcutaneously in abdomen only	Myocardial infarction–anti-coagulant
Epinephrine 1:1,000 for subcutaneous/ IM administration	SQ or IM (preferred): 0.2 to 0.5 mg of 1:1,000 solution; may repeat in 20 minutes	Anaphylaxis and bronchodilator
Epinephrine 1:10,000 IV	IV: 1 mg/10 mL of 1:10,000 solution every 3 to 5 minutes or ET: 2 to 2.5 mg in 10 mL NS	PEA, asystole, pulseless VT, or VF
Epinephrine IV continuous infusion	Adult: 0.1 to 0.5 mcg/kg/min titrate to goal BP	Symptomatic bradycardia, or hypotension/ shock
Esmolol	Bolus: 500 mcg/kg over 1 minute. Initial dose: 50 mcg/kg/min for 4 minutes. Titrate 50 mcg/kg/min every 5 minutes to goal HR/BP. Max: 200 mcg/kg/min	SVT; beta-blocker for HTN emergency Intra/ postoperative tachycardia/HTN

(*continued*)

Medication	Dose	Use
Etomidate (Amidate®)	Initial: 0.3 mg/kg IV (range 0.2 to 0.6 mg/kg)	Moderate sedation for RSI or shoulder reduction
Fentanyl	Bolus: 1 mcg/kg. Initial: 1 mcg/kg/hr. Titrate every 30 minutes. Max: 10 mcg/kg/hr	Narcotic analgesic, sedative
Flumazenil (Romazicon®)	0.2 to 0.5 mg IV over 30 seconds; max cumulative dose: 3 mg	Antidote for benzodiazepine overdose
Fosphenytoin sodium (Cerebyx®)	Load: 15 to 20 phenytoin equivalents per kg by IM or IV 150 mg/min or less	Seizures
Furosemide (Lasix®)	IV: 20 to 40 mg; PO: 20 to 80 mg; higher doses may be administered	Congestive heart failure, edema, hypertension, intracranial pressure
Gentamicin sulfate ophthalmic ointment	0.5-inch ribbon to inside affected lower eyelid	Conjunctivitis and corneal abrasions
Glucagon	0.5 to 2 mg subcutaneous/ IM/IV push	Hypoglycemia, calcium channel or beta-blocker overdose, and esophageal food bolus
Haloperidol lactate (Haldol®)	Adult: 2 to 5 mg IM every 4 to 8 hours as needed	Antipsychotic
Heparin sodium. *Check PTT and guaiac stool before giving*	IV bolus: 60 to 80 unit/kg; max 4,000 units. Then 12 to 18 unit/kg/hr continuous infusion; follow institutional specific protocol.	Anticoagulant for acute myocardial infarction atrial fibrillation, pulmonary embolism, and stroke

(continued)

Medication	Dose	Use
Hydrocodone and acetaminophen (Norco®, Vicodin®)	Adult: hydrocodone 2.5 to 10 mg every 4 to 6 hours as needed for pain; children 2 to 13 years or <50 kg: hydrocodone 0.1 to 0.2 mg/kg/dose every 4 to 6 hours, do *not* exceed six doses per day or acetaminophen max.	Opioid analgesic for pain
Ibuprofen (Motrin®, Advil®)	Infants >6 months and children <12 years: 10 mg/kg/dose PO (max dose 400 mg) every 4 to 6 hrs; Max daily dose 40 mg/kg/d Children 12 to 17 years: 400 mg PO every 4 to 6 hrs; Max daily dose 2,400 mg Adults: 200 to 800 mg every 6 hours as needed for pain; max daily dose 3,200 mg	Analgesic, fever, inflammation (NSAID)
Insulin (regular). *Check blood sugar every hour*	Adult IV varies according to blood sugar: bolus (optional) 0.1 unit/kg, then IV drip according to order and blood sugar. Subcutaneously: 0.5 to 1 unit/kg/d divided into meal time doses	Diabetic ketoacidosis; hyperglycemia
Ipratropium bromide (Atrovent®)	Child: 125 to 250 mcg by nebulizer every 4 to 6 hours. Adult: 500 mcg by nebulizer four times a day. Max: 24 doses in 24 hours	Bronchodilator/anticholinergic for asthma and chronic obstructive pulmonary disease
Labetalol hydrochloride (Normodyne®)	10 to 20 mg IV over 2 minutes, may double dose every 10–15 min as often as necessary; max cumulative dose 300 mg	Hypertension
Levalbuterol hydrochloride (Xopenex®)	Nebulizer: Children 6 to 11 years: 0.31 mg to 0.63 mg. Children ≥12 years and adult: 0.63 to 2.5 mg	Bronchodilator for asthma. Causes less tachycardia than albuterol.
Levofloxacin (Levaquin®). *If given too fast causes arrhythmias*	250 to 750 mg by PO/IV infusion at 500 mg/hr or 750 mg over 1.5 hr	Antibiotic

(*continued*)

Medication	Dose	Use
Lidocaine hydrochloride (Xylocaine®)	IV push: 1 to 1.5 mg/kg, may repeat at 0.5 to 0.75 mg/kg in 5 to 10 minutes. Intravenous drip 1 to 4 mg/min. ET: 2 to 4 mg/kg	Ventricular fibrillation/ ventricular tachycardia. Can be given subcutaneously locally to numb a wound. Comes in 1% or 2% vials.
Lidocaine with epinephrine. *Not for finger/ nose/ears/toes*	Subcutaneously locally 1% or 2% vials	To numb a bleeding wound
Lorazepam (Ativan®)	0.1 mg/kg up to 4 mg IV or IM; 2 to 4 mg by mouth	Seizures, anxiety, and sedation
Magnesium sulfate	Cardiac arrest: 1 to 2 g in 10 mL D_5W or NS over 1 to 2 minutes. If stable: 1 g/50 mL NS over 30 minutes intravenously	Torsades de pointes, hypomagnese- mia, and asthma; smooth muscle relaxant
Mannitol strengths: 5%, 10%, 15%, 20%, and 25%	0.25 to 1 g/kg over 30 to 60 minutes; use inline filter	Intracranial pressure
Meperidine hydrochloride (Demerol®),	Adult: 50 to 100 mg PO, IM, or IV	Opioid analgesic and shiver control
Methotrexate. Use chemotherapy precautions	Adult: 50 mg/m^2 by IM	Miscarriages/ ectopic pregnancy
Methyl- prednisolone (Solu-Medrol®)	Adult 100 to 250 mg IV or IM (average 125 mg)	Steroid to decrease inflammation in asthma; allergic reaction; shock

(*continued*)

Medication	Dose	Use
Metoprolol (Lopressor®)	IV: 2.5 to 5 mg every 2 to 5 min. (max total dose: 15 mg in 15 min.)	Blood pressure, afib/flutter, SVT, and ventricular rate control
Midazolam (Versed®)	Initial intravenous drip: 1 mg/hr. Titrate 1 mg/hr every 15 minutes to achieve sedation goal. Max: 10 mg/hr	Moderate sedation, sedation for mechanically ventilated, or RSI
Morphine sulfate	2 to 5 mg IV over 1 to 5 minutes	Chest pain or pain (opioid analgesic)
Naloxone hydrochloride (Narcan®)	IV, IM, SQ: 0.4 to 2 mg. Max. 10 mg in 10 minutes. Can give via ET tube or nebulizer.	Opiate overdose with respiratory or neurodepression
Nicardipine (Cardene®)	IV initial: 2.5 to 5 mg/hr; titrate every 15 minutes to goal blood pressure; max: 15 mg/hr	Blood pressure
Nitroglycerin (Nitro-Dur, Nitrostat®). *Monitor blood pressure for hypotension; must have intravenous access before giving.*	IV intial: 5 to 20 mcg/min titrate for chest pain/blood pressure by 5 mcg/min every 3 to 5 minutes. Max: 400 mcg/min. Sublingual: one tab every 5 min for a 3-tablet maximum per blood pressure/chest pain	Vasodilator; chest pain; acute myocardial infarction; congestive heart failure; and hypertension
Nitroprusside sodium (Nipride®). *Medicine reacts to light; cover material provided from pharmacy.*	IV: 0.3 to 2 mcg/kg/min titrate up every few minutes until stable blood pressure/chest pain	Hypertension; reduce afterload in congestive heart failure; pulmonary edema; or valve regurgitation

(*continued*)

Medication	Dose	Use
Norepinephrine bitartrate (Levophed®)	Adult: 0.1 to 1 mcg/kg/min titrate to goal BP	Vasopressor for severe shock, drug overdose, or poison-induced hypotension
Oxycodone and acetaminophen (Percocet®)	PO: 2.5 to 10 mg	Opioid analgesic
Phenytoin sodium (Dilantin®). *Infiltration = tissue necrosis, be careful.*	Loading dose: 15 to 20 mg/kg or 1,000 mg IV. *No faster* than 50 mg/min or 20 mg/min in geriatrics	Seizures. *Attach a micron filter.*
Promethazine hydrochloride (Phenergan®)	12.5 to 25 mg by PO, IM, IV, or suppository	Nausea and vomiting
Proparacaine hydrochloride (Alcaine®)	One to two drops to affected eye	To numb the eye. *If used repeatedly, can be corrosive to eye!*
Propofol (Diprivan®)	Initial IV dose: 5 mcg/kg/min. Titrate 5 mcg/kg/min every 5 minutes. Max: 50 mcg/kg/min	Sedation for mechanically ventilated, RSI. *Note:* Check state law for RN administration conditions.
Propranolol hydrochloride (Inderal®)	Adult: 10 to 40 mg PO 2 to 4 times a day. Intravenous bolus: 1 to 3 mg at 1 mg/min; may repeat in 2 minutes.	Hypertension; acute myocardial infarction; dysrhythmias, or thyroid storm
RhoGAM injection	Adult: 300 mcg by injection	Rh-negative pregnant mother

(continued)

Medication	Dose	Use
Sodium bicarbonate	IV bolus: 1 mEq/kg 1 amp = 50 mEq	Acidosis; hyperkalemia; diabetic ketoacidosis; lactic acidosis, and metabolic acidosis
Sodium polystyrene sulfonate (Kayexalate*)	15 to 60 g by mouth or rectally	Removes potassium from body.
Succinyl-choline (Anectine*)	IV: 1.5 mg/kg	Paralytic for intubation. Have ambu bag ready! Causes hyperkalemia and bradycardia.
Tenecteplase (TNKase*)	Weight-based dosing; IV bolus 30 to 50 mg	Thrombolytic (clot buster); STEMI
Tetracaine eyedrops	One to two drops to affected eye	Topical anesthetic to the eye. *Repeated use = eye corrosion!*
Vasopressin (Pitressin*, Vasocrit*)	IV/intraosseous drip: 0.03 units/min. No titration	Vasodilatory shock; catechol-amine sparing vasopressor
Verapamil hydrochloride	Intravenous bolus: 5 to 10 mg over 3 min. May repeat at 10 mg every 30 minutes. Max total dose: 20 mg	PSVT with narrow complex. A-fib or A-flutter
Warfarin sodium (Coumadin*, Jantoven*)	Initial: 2.5 to 5 mg/d; titrate based on INR levels	Anticoagulant

*The definitions of abbreviations can be found in Appendix D.

Appendix C
Critical IV Drips

Fill out formulary kept in your hospital and keep this list in your pocket or with your calculator:

Epinephrine _____mg/_____mL (_____mcg/mL); range: 0.1 to 0.5 mcg/kg/min

Norepinephrine (Levophed®) _____mg/_____mL (_____mcg/mL); range: 0.1 to 1 mcg/kg/min

Dopamine _____mg/_____mL (_____mcg/mL); initial: 5 mcg/kg/min; max = 20 mcg/kg/min

Propofol (Diprivan®) _____mcg/mL; initial: 5 to 10 mcg/kg/min; max: 50 mcg/kg/min

Lidocaine _____G/_____mL (_____mcg/mL); range: 1 to 4 mg/min

Heparin _____units/_____mL (_____units/mL); weight-based hospital-specific protocol

Nitroglycerin _____mg/_____mL (_____mcg/mL); initial: 5 mcg/min; max = 400 mcg/min

Dobutamine _____mg/_____mL (_____mcg/mL); initial: 2.5 mcg/kg/min; max: 40 mcg/kg/min

Nitroprusside (Nipride®) _____mg/_____mL (____mcg/mL); initial: 0.3 to 0.5 mcg/kg/min; max = 2 mcg/kg/min

Amiodarone _____mg/_____mL (_____mg/mL); loading dose: 150 mg over 10 minutes; maintenance dose: 1 mg/min for 6 hours, then 0.5 mg/min for 18 hours

Milrinone _____mg/_____mL (_____mcg/mL); range: 0.375 to 0.75 mcg/kg/min

Midazolam (Versed®) _____mg/_____mL (1 mg/__mL); range: 0.02 to 0.1 mg/kg/hr or 1 to 10 mg/hr

Labetalol _____mg/_____mL (_____mg/mL); initial: 2 mg/min; max cumulative total dose: 300 mg

Diltiazem (Cardizem®) _____mg/_____mL (_____mg/mL); initial: 5 mg/hr; max: 15 mg/hr

Vasopressin _____units/_____mL (_____units/mL); fixed rate: 0.03 units/min for shock

Fentanyl _____mg/_____mL (_____mcg/mL); range: 1 to 10 mcg/kg/hr

Nicardipine (Cardene®) _____mg/_____mL (_____mg/mL); initial: 5 mg/hr; max: 15 mg/hr

Appendix D
Abbreviations

The emergency department nurse must be familiar with many abbreviations, which allow for quicker oral and written communication. For the sake of clarity and readability, terms have been spelled out in the text. Following is the list of common abbreviations for terms used in the text.

abd	abdominal
ABC	airway, breathing, and circulation
ABG	arterial blood gas
ACLS	advanced cardiovascular life support
ADH	antidiuretic hormone
A-fib	atrial fibrillation
A-flutter	atrial flutter
AIDS	acquired immunodeficiency syndrome
ALT/SGPT	alanine aminotransferase/serum glutamic pyruvic transaminase
AMI	acute myocardial infarction
ARDS	acute respiratory distress syndrome
ASAP	as soon as possible
ASD	atrial septal defect

AST/SGOT	aspartate aminotransferase/serum glutamic-oxalo-acetic transaminase
AV	atrioventricular
AVSD	atrioventricular septal defect
b.i.d.	twice daily
BiPAP	bilevel positive airway pressure
BMP	basic metabolic panel
BP	blood pressure
bpm	beats per minute
BRAT	bananas, rice, applesauce, and toast
BS	blood sugar
BSC	bedside commode
BUN	blood urea nitrogen
BVM	bag valve mask
CAD	coronary artery disease
CBC	complete blood count
CDC	Centers for Disease Control and Prevention
CEN	certified emergency nurse
CHD	congenital heart disease
CHF	congestive heart failure
CKMB	creatine kinase MB
CMP	complete metabolic panel
CO_2	carbon dioxide
c/o	complaining of
COPD	chronic obstructive pulmonary disease
CP	chest pain
C-PAP	continuous positive airway pressure
CPR	cardiopulmonary resuscitation
CSF	cerebrospinal fluid
CT	computed tomography
CVA	cerebrovascular accident
DC	discharge

DIB	difficulty in breathing
DIC	disseminated intravascular coagulation
DKA	diabetic ketoacidosis
dx	diagnose
ED	emergency department
EKG	electrocardiogram
EMTALA	Emergency Medical Treatment and Active Labor Act
ENA	Emergency Nurses Association
ENPC	emergency nurse pediatric course
ENT	ear, nose, and throat
ER	emergency room
ESI	Emergency Severity Index
ET	endotracheal tube
ETOH	alcohol
FFP	fresh frozen plasma
FHT	fetal heart tones
FO	foreign object
GCS	Glasgow Coma Scale
GERD	gastroesophageal reflux disease
GI	gastrointestinal
gtts	drops
HA	headache
HCO_3^-	bicarbonate
H_2CO_3	carbonic acid
Hcg	human chorionic gonadotropin
HCT	hematocrit
HGB	hemoglobin
HHNC	hyperosmolar, hyperglycemic nonketotic coma
HHS	hyperosmolar hyperglycemic syndrome
HIV	human immunodeficiency virus
HOB	head of the bed

HPV	human papilloma virus
HTN	hypertension
hx	history
IBS	irritable bowel syndrome
ICP	increased cranial pressure
ICU	intensive care unit
I&D	incision and drainage
IM	intramuscular injection
IMR	intermediate restorative material
INR	international normalized ratio
IO	intraosseous
I&O	intake and output
IUP	intrauterine pregnancy
IV	intravenous
IVC	inferior vena cava
JVD	jugular vein distention
LFT	liver function test
LLQ	left lower quadrant
LOC	loss of consciousness
LP	lumbar puncture
LSD	D-lysergic acid diethylamide
LUQ	left upper quadrant
MDI	meter dose inhaler
MRSA	methicillin-resistant *Staphylococcus aureus*
MS	multiple sclerosis
MVI	multivitamin
NC	nasal cannula
Neb	nebulizer
NG	nasogastric
NIHSS	National Institutes of Health Stroke Scale

NINDS	National Institute for Neurological Disorders and Stroke
NPO	nothing by mouth
NPS	new psychoactive substance
NRB	nonrebreather
NRP	Neonatal Resuscitation Program
NS	normal saline
NSAID	nonsteroidal anti-inflammatory drug
NTG	nitrogylcerine
NVD	nausea/vomiting/diarrhea
O_2	oxygen
OD	overdose
OM	otitis media
OR	operating room
os	opening
$PaCO_2$	partial pressure of carbon dioxide
PALS	pediatric advanced life support
PDA	patent ductus arteriosus
PE	pulmonary embolism
PEA	pulseless electrical activity
PEEP	positive end-expiratory pressure
PID	pelvic inflammatory disease
PIH	pregnancy-induced hypertension
PLT	platelets
PO	by mouth
PPE	personal protective equipment
pr	by rectum
PRBC	packed red blood cells
prn	as needed
PSVT	paroxysmal supraventricular tachycardia
pt.	patient

PT	prothrombin time
PTT	partial thromboplastin time
PTU	propylthiouracil
PVC	premature ventricular contraction
PVD	peripheral vascular disease
RBC	red blood cell
resp	respiratory
RF	renal failure
RL	Ringer's lactate
RLQ	right lower quadrant
ROM	range of motion
RSI	rapid sequence intubation
RSV	respiratory syncytial virus
RUQ	right upper quadrant
SANE	sexual assault nurse examiner
SC	subcutaneous
SIADH	syndrome of inappropriate antidiuretic hormone
SIDS	sudden infant death syndrome
SIRS	systemic inflammatory response syndrome
SL	under the tongue
SOB	shortness of breath
s/s	signs and symptoms
stat	immediately
STD	sexually transmitted disease
SVT	supraventricular tachycardia
SZ	seizure
TB	tuberculosis
Tdap	tetanus diphtheria and pertussis
TIA	transient ischemic attack
TNCC	trauma nurse core course
tPA	tissue plasminogen activator

TSS	toxic shock syndrome
Tx	treat or treatment
UA	urinalysis
US	ultrasound
UTI	urinary tract infection
VF	ventricular fibrillation
VS	vital signs
VSD	ventricular septal defect
VT	ventricular tachycardia

Appendix E
12-Lead EKGs and
Common Dysrhythmias

PROPER EKG LEAD PLACEMENT

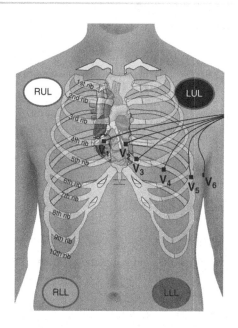

Limb leads may be placed symmetrically on the upper and lower extremities on a nonbony surface.

BREAKDOWN OF NORMAL SINUS RHYTHM

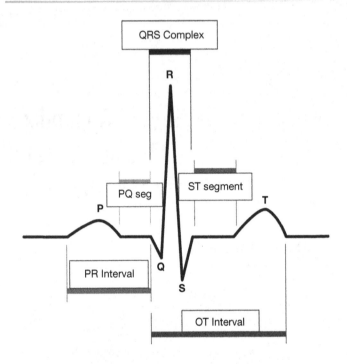

P wave represents: contraction and depolarization of the atria.

QRS complex: represents contraction and depolarization of the ventricles.

T wave represents: ventricular relaxation, repolarization, and passive filling.

OTHER COMMON EKG RHYTHMS

Normal Sinus Rhythm

Note P wave for every QRS complex. Rate is regular.

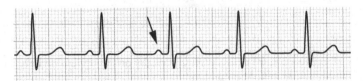

Atrial Fibrillation

Note atrial rhythm waves, P wave unidentifiable, and irregular rate.

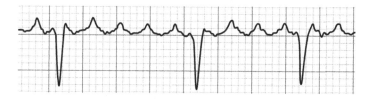

Atrial Flutter

Note multiple-peaked or saw-tooth-like P waves.

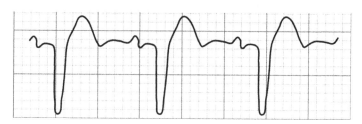

Left Bundle Branch Block

Note wide QRS > 0.12 seconds.

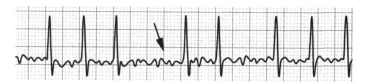

First-Degree Block

Note rate is regular and the PR interval is longer or >0.20 seconds.

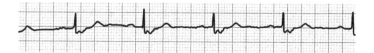

Second-Degree Heart Block, Mobitz Type I, or Wenckebach

Note irregular yet patterned rate. See how PR interval becomes progressively longer until finally a QRS complex is dropped.

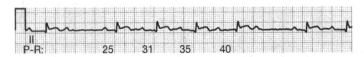

| P-R: | 25 | 31 | 35 | 40 |

Second-Degree Heart Block, Mobitz Type II

The PR interval does not progressively lengthen, but a QRS complex gets dropped regularly.

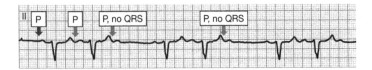

Third-Degree or (Complete) Heart Block

The P waves occur at regular intervals and the QRS complexes occur at regular intervals but they are disconnected and do not occur together. This is due to a complete electrical blockage between the atria (p wave) and the ventricles (QRS complex).

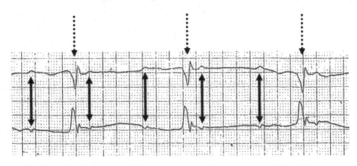

Paced or Ventricular Paced Rhythm

Note pacer spikes instead of P waves.

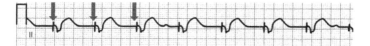

Wolff Parkinsons White Syndrome

Note the delta wave in the upstroke of the QRS complex.

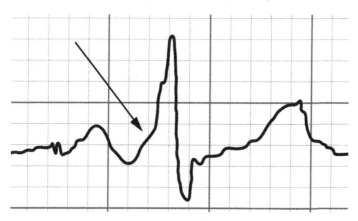

Torsades de Pointes

Torsades de pointes is French for "turning or twisting of the points." Note that this particular type of ventricular tachycardia turns or twists on its axis much like a strand of DNA. The treatment for this type of tachycardia is magnesium sulfate.

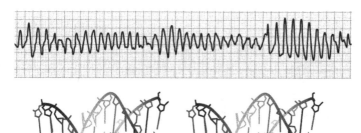

Junctional

Note there are either no P waves present or the P waves are inverted.

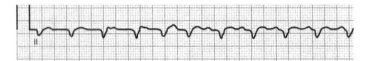

Premature Atrial Contraction

Note that the underlying rate is regular except for an occasional early narrow complex beat.

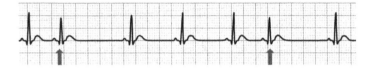

Premature Ventricular Contraction

Note that the underlying rate is regular with an occasional wide complex beat.

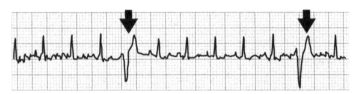

Bigeminy

Note the premature ventricular contraction (PVC) with every other beat.

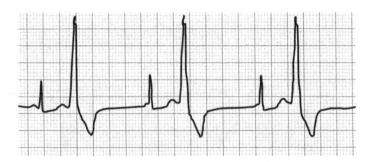

Couplet

Note two PVCs in a row.

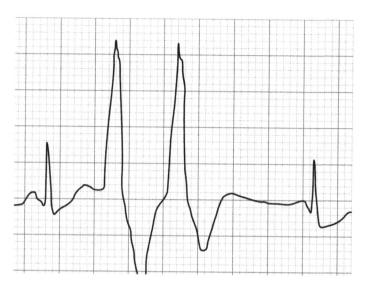

Appendix F
Skills Check-Off Sheets

Employee Name _____

Start Date _____

ITEM/SKILL For day 1 of orientation (no patient assignment)	Verbally reviewed	Physically demonstrated	Preceptor initials
Assistance notification: (supervisor, security, chaplain, Division of Family and Children Services, case/risk management, ethics committee, sheriff)			
Call-in policy			
Clock-in/clock-out procedures			
Communication books and boards			
Discuss orientation needs and establish goals			
Education resources/requirements/ opportunities			
Employee occurrence reports			
EMTALA guidelines			
Intercom/patient call light system			

(continued)

ITEM/SKILL For day 1 of orientation (no patient assignment)	Verbally reviewed	Physically demonstrated	Preceptor initials
Latex allergy protocol and procedures			
Manual time record			
Medication adverse reaction form or procedure			
Medication occurrence report			
Medication administration (PO/IM/IV)			
Nursing documentation forms			
Nursing/ED policy and procedure manual			
Orient to unit/staff personnel/ registration			
Orientation forms and packet			
Orientation schedule			
Patient-appropriate room assignments			
Patient assignment board procedures			
Patient belongings left in department			
Patient education resources			
Patient flow in department			
Patient occurrence report			
Reference manuals			
Registration process			
Scavenger hunt			
Schedule/request form for time off/PTO			
Staffing assignments			
Storeroom supplies			
Supply stocking procedure			
Telephone system			

(continued)

ITEM/SKILL For day 1 of orientation (no patient assignment)	Verbally reviewed	Physically demonstrated	Preceptor initials
Time and attendance policy			
Tour of department			
Videos to watch:			

ITEM/SKILL Week 1, nonurgent patient assignment Review Chapters 1, 4, 17, 18	Verbally reviewed	Physically demonstrated	Preceptor initials
Accu-chek machine and documentation			
Animal bite protocols			
Blanket warmer purpose and use			
Burn care procedures			
Care of patients assigned to nonurgent areas			
Computer systems/sign-up for classes			
Crash cart/Braslow cart locations			
Dermabond administration			
Diagnostic tests (x-ray, CT scan, MRI, VQ scan, US)			
Difficult people, working with them			
Discharge procedures and instructions			
Ear irrigation/Morgan eye lens			
Evaluation form, reassess goals weekly			
Eye exams supplies: Wood's lamp, eye kit, slit lamp			

(continued)

ITEM/SKILL Week 1, nonurgent patient assignment Review Chapters 1, 4, 17, 18	Verbally reviewed	Physically demonstrated	Preceptor initials
Immobilization and splinting techniques (Ortho-Glass)			
Incision and drainage procedures			
Instrument recycling (disposable/nondisposable)			
Joint commission information			
Language translation methods (verbal/written)			
Minor or urgent care policies and procedures			
Medication administration policies and procedures			
Pain assessment and documentation			
Pain management policy/procedures			
Positioning and securing of pediatric patient (papoose)			
Rapid strep screen collection procedure			
Respiratory aerosol nebulizer treatment			
Safety data sheets (SDS)			
Supplies for nonurgent care areas			
Suture/staple removal procedure			
Suture/wound care supplies, protocols, techniques			
Tetanus prophylaxis			
Treatment of minors in the ED			
Urine collection procedures			
Use/purpose of soiled utility room			

(continued)

ITEM/SKILL **Week 1, nonurgent patient assignment** Review Chapters 1, 4, 17, 18	Verbally reviewed	Physically demonstrated	Preceptor initials
Use/purpose/flow of patients in minor or urgent care department			
Visual acuity (adult or pediatric)			
Worker's compensation drug screening			

ITEM/SKILL **Weeks 2–4, nonurgent patient and pelvic room assignment** Review Chapters 7, 8, 9, 10, 11, 16	Verbally reviewed	Physically demonstrated	Preceptor initials
Abuse/neglect evaluation			
AMA (patient leaving against medical advice) procedures			
Assessments: primary, secondary, focused			
BEAR hugger or warming blanket uses/purposes			
Blood work interpretation			
Care of nonurgent patients			
C-spine immobilization and removal techniques			
Documentation of assessment/treatment/medication			
Doppler: vessel and obstetric uses			
EMS radio and H.E.A.R. system radio			
Evaluation form, reassess goals weekly			
Fetal heart monitoring in ED			
Finger traps			
Foley catheter removal			

(continued)

ITEM/SKILL Weeks 2–4, nonurgent patient and pelvic room assignment Review Chapters 7, 8, 9, 10, 11, 16	Verbally reviewed	Physically demonstrated	Preceptor initials
Foley catheterization, urine meter			
GYN exam/specimens and products of conception			
Head lamp			
IV insertion (INT) procedures			
IV infusion pumps			
Left without treatment procedures			
Methotrexate for ectopic pregnancy			
Miscarriage (complete/incomplete) referrals			
Morgan eye lens/eye irrigation techniques			
Nonurgent patient acuity			
Nosebleed procedures and equipment			
Pain assessment and documentation			
Patient teaching documentation			
Pelvic stretchers			
Pelvic supplies			
Phlebotomy check-off, venipunctures lab, and IV access			
Portable monitor systems			
Precipitous delivery procedures and supplies			
Rape/sexual assault examination protocol			
Rapid flu specimen collection			
RhoGAM/blood product administration			

(continued)

ITEM/SKILL Weeks 2–4, nonurgent patient and pelvic room assignment Review Chapters 7, 8, 9, 10, 11, 16	Verbally reviewed	Physically demonstrated	Preceptor initials
Respiratory syncytial virus specimen collection (RSV)			
Stool specimen collection			
Urinary catheterization procedures, Quik cath (8fr, 5fr)			
Urology cart/supplies			
Use/purpose/flow in the nonurgent rooms			
Vital sign monitoring of nonurgent patients			

ITEM/SKILL Weeks 5–8, urgent patient assignment Review Chapters 2, 6, 12, 13, 14, 19, 20	Verbally reviewed	Physically demonstrated	Preceptor initials
(Suicidal/homicidal) forms			
12-Lead EKG check-off and interpretation			
Acute allergic reaction (anaphylaxis)			
Admission procedure			
Advance directives and do not resuscitate (DNR) status			
Airway open/maintain: nontrauma and trauma			
Airway/breathing supplies and usage in ED			
Anesthesia consent			
Arterial blood gas interpretation			

(*continued*)

ITEM/SKILL Weeks 5–8, urgent patient assignment Review Chapters 2, 6, 12, 13, 14, 19, 20	Verbally reviewed	Physically demonstrated	Preceptor initials
Bag valve mask: adult, pediatric, neonatal			
Blood/blood products administration and forms			
Central port access (gripper/Huber needle)			
Central vein access kit and procedures			
Crash cart, Braslow cart			
Endotracheal intubation and rapid-sequence intubation			
Evaluation form, reassess goals weekly			
Gastric lavage/Lavacuator tube, NG tube (oral/nasal)			
GI bleed procedures			
Hare traction splint			
Hemoccult/stool/gastric specimen collection			
Holding of admitted patients			
Lumbar puncture tray, procedure/patient position			
Mental health patient care			
Monitoring system: central, bedside, portable			
Neonate patient care			
Neutropenia policy and procedures			
OR admission and preoperative checklist			
Patient transfer procedure and transfer			

(continued)

ITEM/SKILL Weeks 5–8, urgent patient assignment Review Chapters 2, 6, 12, 13, 14, 19, 20	Verbally reviewed	Physically demonstrated	Preceptor initials
Pediatric care and reference manuals			
Peritoneal lavage			
Purpose/use/flow of urgent room assignments			
Respiratory care check-off			
Seclusion/restraint policy			
Secondary assessments and reassessments			
Security policy regarding mental health patients			
Sedation and analgesia policy and procedures/forms			
Sputum specimen collection procedures			
Surgical consent			
Tuberculosis suspected patient care			
Urgent patient acuity			
Urgent patient supplies			
Ventilator troubleshooting and patient care			

ITEM/SKILL Weeks 9–12, priority 1 emergent patient and triage assignment Review Chapters 3, 5, 15, 21, 22, 23	Verbally reviewed	Physically demonstrated	Preceptor initials
ACLS and PALS protocols			
Biphasic defibrillator			
Cardiac arrhythmias			

(continued)

ITEM/SKILL Weeks 9–12, priority 1 emergent patient and triage assignment Review Chapters 3, 5, 15, 21, 22, 23	Verbally reviewed	Physically demonstrated	Preceptor initials
Chest tube equipment/procedures: hemo/pneumothorax			
Code blue form and code blue critique form			
Code blue procedure in the ED			
Code blue procedures out of the ED			
Crash cart			
Cricothyrotomy kit and procedure			
Death in the department/physician pronouncements			
Deceased patient data form			
Decontamination equipment			
Defibrillator/pacer procedures			
Disaster plan			
Emergency medications and resource manual			
Emergent acuity patients			
Emergent patient supplies			
ED nurse's role in cardiopulmonary arrest			
Evaluation form and revise goals weekly			
Heimlich valve			
Infusion protocols (cardiac/emergency infusions)			
Level 1 rapid infuser/fluid warming equipment/supplies			
Multiple trauma patient care			
Needle decompression			

(continued)

ITEM/SKILL Weeks 9–12, priority 1 emergent patient and triage assignment Review Chapters 3, 5, 15, 21, 22, 23	Verbally reviewed	Physically demonstrated	Preceptor initials
Neurological assessment/ documentation			
Patient priority setting			
Pericardiocentesis tray			
Pervenous temporary pacemaker			
Poison control notification/ documentation			
Pregnant trauma patient care			
Seizure precautions and patient care			
Tackle boxes for tPA, allergy, transport, TNKase, rapid sequence intubation			
Therapeutic hypothemia protocol			
TPA/TNKase policies/procedures: acute MI, stroke			
Tracheostomy tray and procedure			
Transcutaneous pacemaker procedure			
Transport defibrillator procedures			
Transport of critical patient			
Triage guidelines/protocols (disaster and nondisaster)			
Use/purpose/flow priority 1 or trauma rooms			
Complete postorientation evaluation form, assessment of the clinical orientation process, review goals, and assess need for orientation extension			

Preceptor Name/Initials: _____

Orientation End Date: _____

Bibliography

American Heart Association. (2016). *Advanced cardiovascular life support.* Dallas, TX: Author.

American Medical Association. (2012). *Basic disaster life support version 3.0.* Chicago, IL: Author.

Armstrong, J. H., & Schwartz, R. B. (2011). *Advanced disaster life support version 3.0.* Chicago, IL: American Medical Association.

Basile, J., & Bloch, M. J. (2014, November 18). Overview of hypertension in adults. Retrieved from http://www.uptodate.com/contents/overview-of -hypertension-in-adults?source=search_result&search=hypertension&s electedTitle=1~150

Blank, F. S., Miller, M., Nichols, J., Smithline, H., Crabb, G., & Pekow, P. (2009). Blood glucose measurement in patients with suspected diabetic ketoacidosis: A comparison of Abbott MediSense PCx point-of-care meter values to reference laboratory values. *Journal of Emergency Nursing, 35,* 93–96. doi:10.1016/j.jen.2008.01.008

Bowen, P. (2016). Early identification, rapid response, and effective treatment of acute stroke: Utilizing teleneurolgoy to ensure optimal clinical outcomes. *MEDSURG Nursing, 25*(4), 241–243.

Centers for Disease Control and Prevention. (2015, April 25). Ebola (Ebola virus disease). Retrieved from http://www.cdc.gov/vhf/ebola/diagnosis/ index.html

Chameides, L., Samson, R. A., Schexnayder, S. M., & Hazinski, M. F. (2016). *Pediatric advanced life support.* Dallas, TX: American Heart Association.

Derr, P., McEvoy, M., & Tardiff, J. (2014). *Emergency & critical care pocket guide* (8th ed.). Burlington, MA: Jones & Bartlett.

Emergency Nurses Association. (2007). *Emergency nursing core curriculum* (6th ed.). Philadelphia, PA: Saunders.

Emergency Nurses Association. (2009). *CEN review manual* (4th ed.). Dubuque, IA: Kendall Hunt.

Emergency Nurses Association. (2012). *Emergency nursing pediatric course* (4th ed.). Des Plaines, IL: Author.

Emergency Nurses Association. (2013). *Sheehy's manual of emergency care* (7th ed.). B. B. Hammond, & P. G. Zimmermann (Eds.). St. Louis, MO: Elsevier Mosby.

Emergency Nurses Association. (2014). *Trauma nurse core course* (7th ed.). Des Plaines, IL: Author.

Gasparis Vonfrolio, L. (1999). *The one and only CEN review course*. Staten Island, NY: Education Enterprises.

Gilboy, N., Tanabe, P., Travers, D., & Roseenau, A. (2012). *Emergency Severity Index (ESI) version 4*. Rockville, MD: Agency for Healthcare Research and Quality.

Goldsworthy, S., & Graham, L. (2014). *Compact clinical guide to mechanical ventilation*. New York, NY: Springer Publishing.

Gupta, A. G., & Adler, M. D. (2016). Management of an unexpected delivery in the emergency department. *Clinical Pediatric Emergency Medicine*, *17*(2), 89–98. doi:10.1016/j.cpem.2016.03.002

Hamilton, R. J. (2016). *Tarascon pocket pharmacopoeia* (30th ed.). Burlington, MA: Jones & Bartlett.

Mader, S. S., & Windelspecht, M. (2016). *Biology* (12th ed.). New York, NY: McGraw-Hill.

National Institutes of Health. (2014, September 8). *Evidence-based management of sickle cell disease: Expert Panel Report, 2014*. Retrieved from http://www.nhlbi.nih.gov/health-pro/guidelines/sickle-cell-disease-guidelines

Nevid, J. S., Rathus, S. A., & Greene, B. (2014). *Abnormal psychology* (9th ed.). Upper Saddle River, NJ: Pearson.

Niermeyer, S. (2015). From the Neonatal Resuscitation Program to Helping Babies Breathe: Global impact of educational programs in neonatal resuscitation. *Seminars in Fetal and Neonatal Medicine*, *20*, 300–308. doi:10.1016/j.siny.2015.06.005

Office of Public Health Preparedness and Response. (2015, November 18). *Emergency preparedness and response*. Retrieved from https://emergency.cdc.gov/bioterrorism/

Opioid overdose prevention toolkit. (2016). Rockville, MD: Department of Health and Human Services, Substance Abuse and Mental Health Services Administration, 2016.

Pagana, K. D., & Pagana, T. J. (2013). St. *Mosby's manual of diagnostic and laboratory tests* (11th ed.). St. Louis, MO: Elsevier Mosby.

Porth, C. M. (2015). *Essentials of pathophysiology* (4th ed.). Philadelphia, PA: Wolters Kluwer.

Prosser, J., & Nelson, L. (2012). The toxicology of bath salts: A review of synthetic cathinones. *Journal of Medical Toxicology*, *8*(1), 33–42. doi:10.1007/s13181-011-0193-z

Shepherd, S. M., & Shoff, W. H. (2014). An urban northeastern United States alligator bite. *American Journal of Emergency Medicine*, *32*(5), 487.e1–487.e3. doi:10.1016/j.ajem.2013.11.004

Visser, L. S., Montejano, A. S., & Grossman, V. A. (2015). *Fast facts for the triage nurse*. New York, NY: Springer Publishing.

Wiegand, T. (2016). Nonsteroidal anti-inflammatory drug (NSAID) toxicity treatment & management. Retrieved from http://emedicine.medscape.com/article/816117-treatment

Wolters Kluwer Clinical Drug Information, Inc. (2016). Lexi Drugs, 2.4.0. Retrieved from http://online.lexi.com/action/home

Index

Page numbers followed by "*f*" indicate a figure; and those followed by "*t*" indicate a table.

REVOLUTIONIZE YOUR ER NURSING ORIENTATION

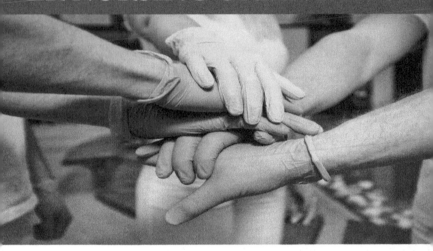

WITH THE INSTRUCTOR TOOLKIT
FOR *FAST FACTS FOR THE ER NURSE*

The ER is a fast-paced department that requires a very distinct set of skills, making orientation a critical and often overwhelming time for new nurses. Don't miss our companion package to this best-selling pocket manual with key teaching elements for the orientation period including:

PowerPoint Presentations
Assignments
Instructor Resource

LEARN MORE TODAY!
VISIT WWW.SPRINGERPUB.COM/9780826126573

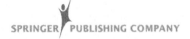

Printed in the United States
By Bookmasters